MAYO CLINIC
CRITICAL CARE
CASE REVIEW

MAYO CLINIC CRITICAL CARE CASE REVIEW

EDITORS

Rahul Kashyap, MBBS
Senior Clinical Research Coordinator,
Department of Anesthesiology,
Mayo Clinic, Rochester, Minnesota
Assistant Professor of Anesthesiology
Mayo Clinic College of Medicine

John C. O'Horo, MD, MPH
Fellow in Infectious Diseases,
Mayo School of Graduate Medical Education and
Assistant Professor of Medicine
Mayo Clinic College of Medicine
Rochester, Minnesota

J. Christopher Farmer, MD
Chair, Department of Critical Care Medicine,
Mayo Clinic, Scottsdale, Arizona
Professor of Medicine
Mayo Clinic College of Medicine

ASSOCIATE EDITORS

Kianoush B. Kashani, MD
James A. Onigkeit, MD
Kannan Ramar, MBBS, MD

MAYO CLINIC SCIENTIFIC PRESS   OXFORD UNIVERSITY PRESS

Contents

SECTION I: CASES

1. **Dyspnea and Edema**   2
   Blair D. Westerly, MD, and Hiroshi Sekiguchi, MD

2. **An Electrical Problem**   6
   Ronaldo A. Sevilla Berrios, MD, and Erica D. Wittwer, MD, PhD

3. **Hypertension**   10
   *Srikant Nannapaneni, MBBS, Lisbeth Y. Garcia Arguello, MD,
   and John G. Park, MD*

4. **A Rare Cause of Liver Failure**   14
   *Alice Gallo de Moraes, MD, Sarah A. Narotzky, MD,
   and Teng Moua, MD*

5. **Shortness of Breath**   18
   Carlos J. Racedo Africano, MD, and Darlene R. Nelson, MD

6. **Acute Respiratory Failure in a Young Smoker**   22
   Mazen O. Al-Qadi, MBBS, and Bernardo J. Selim, MD

7. **Shock**   26
   *Mazen O. Al-Qadi, MBBS, John C. O'Horo, MD, MPH,
   and Larry M. Baddour, MD*

8. Diffuse Abdominal Pain in a 45-Year-Old Woman 32
Mazen O. Al-Qadi, MBBS, Jasleen R. Pannu, MBBS,
and Teng Moua, MD

9. An Over-the-Counter Intoxication 36
Ronaldo A. Sevilla Berrios, MD, and Kianoush B. Kashani, MD

10. An Over-the-Counter Overdose 42
Mazen O. Al-Qadi, MBBS, Sarah B. Nelson, PharmD, RPh,
and Bernardo J. Selim, MD

11. A Post–Myocardial Infarction Complication 48
Mazen O. Al-Qadi, MBBS, and Eric L. Bloomfield, MD

12. Massive Hemoptysis 52
Mazen O. Al-Qadi, MBBS, and Mark E. Wylam, MD

13. Hypotension Following a Broken Hip 58
Joseph H. Skalski, MD, and Daryl J. Kor, MD

14. Extubation Failure 62
Muhammad A. Rishi, MBBS, and Nathan J. Smischney, MD

15. Hypotension and Right-Sided Heart Failure After Left Pneumonectomy 66
Misty A. Radosevich, MD, W. Brian Beam, MD, and Onur Demirci, MD

16. More Than Meets the Eye 70
Sumedh S. Hoskote, MBBS, Shivani S. Shinde, MBBS,
and Nathan J. Smischney, MD

17. Reverse Apical Ballooning Syndrome Due to Clonidine Withdrawal 74
Pramod K. Guru, MBBS, Dereddi Raja S. Reddy, MD,
and Nandan S. Anavekar, MB, BCh

18. A Well-Known Cardiac Condition With a Unique Presentation 80
Sumedh S. Hoskote, MBBS, Muhammad A. Rishi, MBBS,
and Nathan J. Smischney, MD

19. Electrolyte Abnormalities During Continuous Renal
Replacement Therapy 84
Sumedh S. Hoskote, MBBS, Fouad T. Chebib, MD,
and Nathan J. Smischney, MD

20. A Disease Masquerading as Septic Shock   90
Muhammad A. Rishi, MBBS, and Nathan J. Smischney, MD

21. A Respiratory Infection   94
Kelly A. Cawcutt, MD, and Cassie C. Kennedy, MD

22. Infection in a Patient With Chronic Myeloid Leukemia   98
Michelle Biehl, MD, Lisbeth Y. Garcia Arguello, MD,
and Teng Moua, MD

23. Torsades de Pointes   104
Andrea B. Johnson, APRN, CNP, and Thomas B. Comfere, MD

24. The Kidneys Can See When the Eyes Cannot   108
Sarah J. Lee, MD, MPH, and Floranne C. Ernste, MD

25. An Upper Airway Crisis   114
Mazen O. Al-Qadi, MBBS, and Mark T. Keegan, MD

26. An Endocrine Emergency   118
W. Brian Beam, MD, and Ognjen Gajic, MD

27. Acute Renal Failure   124
Mazen O. Al-Qadi, MBBS, and Amy W. Williams, MD

28. Hypoxia and Diffuse Pulmonary Infiltrates in
an Immunosuppressed Patient With Vasculitis   130
Matthew E. Nolan, MD, and Ulrich Specks, MD

29. A Paraneoplastic Syndrome   136
Andres Borja Alvarez, MD, and Emir Festic, MD

30. Complicated Diarrheal Illness   142
Arjun Gupta, MBBS, and Sahil Khanna, MBBS

31 Persistent Shock With Hemorrhagic Complications   146
Sangita Trivedi, MBBS, Rahul Kashyap, MBBS,
and Michael E. Nemergut, MD, PhD

32. An Unusual Presentation of Disseminated Histoplasmosis   150
Lokendra Thakur, MBBS, and Vivek Iyer, MD, MPH

33. Complications of Cirrhosis   154
Raina Shivashankar, MD, and Purna C. Kashyap, MBBS

34. A Curious Case of Abdominal Pain   158
*Pramod K. Guru, MBBS, Abbasali Akhoundi, MD,
and Kianoush B. Kashani, MD*

35. Weakness in the Intensive Care Unit   162
Christopher L. Kramer, MD, and Alejandro A. Rabinstein, MD

36. Altered Mental Status and Rigidity   166
Christopher L. Kramer, MD, and Alejandro A. Rabinstein, MD

37. Overdose   170
Arjun Gupta, MBBS, and Sahil Khanna, MBBS

38. An Unusual Encephalopathy   174
Rudy M. Tedja, DO, and Teng Moua, MD

39. Brain Death   178
*Dereddi Raja S. Reddy, MD, Sudhir V. Datar, MBBS,
and Eelco F. M. Wijdicks, MD, PhD*

40. Use of Extracorporeal Membrane Oxygenation
for Acute Respiratory Distress Syndrome   184
Kelly A. Cawcutt, MD, Craig E. Daniels, MD, and Gregory J. Schears, MD

41. Chest Pain and Respiratory Distress   190
David W. Barbara, MD, and William J. Mauermann, MD

42. Portal Venous Gas   194
*Brendan T. Wanta, MD, Arun Subramanian, MBBS,
and Mark T. Keegan, MD*

43. Acute Respiratory Failure in a Stem Cell Transplant Patient   198
Channing C. Twyner, MD, and Arun Subramanian, MBBS

44. Flail Chest   202
*Sumedh S. Hoskote, MBBS, John C. O'Horo, MD, MPH,
and Craig E. Daniels, MD*

45. Coma 206
Muhammad A. Rishi, MBBS, Sarah J. Lee, MD, MPH,
and Teng Moua, MD

46. A Bleeding Disorder 210
John C. O'Horo, MD, MPH, and Philippe R. Bauer, MD, PhD

47. A Cardiopulmonary Resuscitation Complication 214
John C. O'Horo, MD, MPH, Sumedh S. Hoskote, MBBS,
and Hiroshi Sekiguchi, MD

48. Severe Influenza A–Associated Acute Respiratory Distress Syndrome 218
Rudy M. Tedja, DO, and Craig E. Daniels, MD

49. Severe Chest Pain 224
Ronaldo A. Sevilla Berrios, MD, and R. Thomas Tilbury, MD

50. A More Frequent Airway Emergency 228
Shihab H. Sugeir, MD, and Francis T. Lytle, MD

SECTION II: QUESTIONS AND ANSWERS

51. Review Questions and Answers 234

Index 279

Contributors

Abbasali Akhoundi, MD
Research Fellow in Nephrology,
Mayo School of Graduate
    Medical Education,
Mayo Clinic College of Medicine,
Rochester, Minnesota

Mazen O. Al-Qadi, MBBS
Fellow in Pulmonary
    and Critical Care Medicine,
Mayo School of Graduate
    Medical Education,
Mayo Clinic College of Medicine,
Rochester, Minnesota

Nandan S. Anavekar, MB, BCh
Consultant,
Division of Cardiovascular Diseases,
Mayo Clinic, Rochester, Minnesota;
Assistant Professor,
Mayo Clinic College of Medicine,
Rochester, Minnesota;

Larry M. Baddour, MD
Chair, Division of Infectious Diseases,
Mayo Clinic, Rochester, Minnesota;
Professor of Medicine,
Mayo Clinic College of Medicine,
Rochester, Minnesota

David W. Barbara, MD
Senior Associate Consultant,
Department of Anesthesiology,
Mayo Clinic, Rochester, Minnesota;
Assistant Professor of Anesthesiology,
Mayo Clinic College of Medicine,
Rochester, Minnesota

Philippe R. Bauer, MD, PhD
Consultant,
Division of Pulmonary and Critical
    Care Medicine,
Mayo Clinic, Rochester, Minnesota;
Associate Professor of Medicine,
Mayo Clinic College of Medicine,
Rochester, Minnesota

W. Brian Beam, MD
Resident in Critical Care
    Medicine, Mayo School of
    Graduate
    Medical Education,
Mayo Clinic College of Medicine,
Rochester, Minnesota

Michelle Biehl, MD
Fellow in Pulmonary
    and Critical Care Medicine,
Mayo School of Graduate
    Medical Education,
Mayo Clinic College of Medicine,
Rochester, Minnesota

Eric L. Bloomfield, MD
Consultant,
Department of Anesthesiology,
Mayo Clinic, Rochester, Minnesota;
Associate Professor of Anesthesiology,
Mayo Clinic College of Medicine,
Rochester, Minnesota

Andres Borja Alvarez, MD
Resident in Pulmonary
    and Critical Care Medicine,
Mayo School of Graduate
    Medical Education,
Mayo Clinic College of Medicine,
Jacksonville, Florida

Kelly A. Cawcutt, MD
Resident in Infectious Diseases,
Mayo School of Graduate
    Medical Education,
Mayo Clinic College of Medicine,
Rochester, Minnesota

Fouad T. Chebib, MD
Fellow in Nephrology,
Mayo School of Graduate
    Medical Education,
Mayo Clinic College of Medicine,
Rochester, Minnesota

Thomas B. Comfere, MD
Consultant,
Department of Anesthesiology,
Mayo Clinic, Rochester, Minnesota;
Assistant Professor of Anesthesiology,
Mayo Clinic College of Medicine,
Rochester, Minnesota

Craig E. Daniels, MD
Consultant,
Division of Pulmonary
    and Critical Care Medicine,
Mayo Clinic, Rochester, Minnesota;
Associate Professor of Medicine,
Mayo Clinic College of Medicine,
Rochester, Minnesota

Sudhir V. Datar, MBBS
Fellow in Critical Care Neurology,
Mayo School of Graduate
    Medical Education,
Mayo Clinic College of Medicine,
Rochester, Minnesota

Onur Demirci, MD
Senior Associate Consultant,
Department of Anesthesiology,
Mayo Clinic, Rochester, Minnesota;
Instructor in Anesthesiology,
Mayo Clinic College of Medicine,
Rochester, Minnesota

Floranne C. Ernste, MD
Consultant,
Division of Rheumatology,
Mayo Clinic, Rochester, Minnesota;
Assistant Professor of Medicine,
Mayo Clinic College of Medicine,
Rochester, Minnesota

Emir Festic, MD
Consultant,
Division of Critical Care Medicine,
Mayo Clinic, Jacksonville, Florida;
Associate Professor of Medicine,
Mayo Clinic College of Medicine,
Rochester, Minnesota

Ognjen Gajic, MD
Consultant,
Division of Pulmonary and Critical
    Care Medicine,
Mayo Clinic, Rochester, Minnesota;
Professor of Medicine,
Mayo Clinic College of Medicine,
Rochester, Minnesota

Alice Gallo de Moraes, MD
Resident in Pulmonary
    and Critical Care Medicine,
Mayo School of Graduate
    Medical Education,
Mayo Clinic College of Medicine,
Rochester, Minnesota

Lisbeth Garcia Arguello, MD
Research Fellow in Pulmonary
    and Critical Care Medicine,
Mayo School of Graduate
    Medical Education,
Mayo Clinic College of Medicine,
Rochester, Minnesota

Arjun Gupta, MBBS
Research Associate,
Division of Infectious Diseases,
Mayo Clinic, Rochester, Minnesota

Pramod K. Guru, MBBS
Fellow in Pulmonary
    and Critical Care Medicine,
Mayo School of Graduate Medical
    Education and Instructor of
    Medicine,
Mayo Clinic College of Medicine,
Rochester, Minnesota

Sumedh S. Hoskote, MBBS
Fellow in Pulmonary
    and Critical Care Medicine,
Mayo School of Graduate Medical
    Education and Assistant
    Professor of Medicine,
Mayo Clinic College of Medicine,
Rochester, Minnesota

Vivek Iyer, MD, MPH
Consultant,
Division of Pulmonary and Critical
    Care Medicine,
Mayo Clinic, Rochester, Minnesota;
Assistant Professor of Medicine,
Mayo Clinic College of Medicine,
Rochester, Minnesota

Andrea B. Johnson, APRN, CNP
Nurse Practitioner,
Critical Care Multidisciplinary
    Program,
Mayo Clinic, Rochester, Minnesota

Kianoush B. Kashani, MD
Consultant,
Division of Nephrology
    and Hypertension,
Mayo Clinic, Rochester, Minnesota;
Assistant Professor of Medicine,
Mayo Clinic College of Medicine,
Rochester, Minnesota

Purna C. Kashyap, MBBS
Consultant,
Division of Gastroenterology
    and Hepatology,
Mayo Clinic, Rochester, Minnesota;
Assistant Professor of Medicine,
Mayo Clinic College of Medicine,
Rochester, Minnesota

Rahul Kashyap, MBBS
Senior Clinical Research Coordinator,
Department of Anesthesiology,
Mayo Clinic, Rochester, Minnesota;
Assistant Professor of Anesthesiology,
Mayo Clinic College of Medicine,
Rochester, Minnesota

Mark T. Keegan, MD
Consultant,
Department of Anesthesiology,
Mayo Clinic, Rochester, Minnesota;
Professor of Anesthesiology,
Mayo Clinic College of Medicine,
Rochester, Minnesota

Cassie C. Kennedy, MD
Consultant,
Division of Pulmonary and Critical
    Care Medicine,
Mayo Clinic, Rochester, Minnesota;
Assistant Professor of Medicine,
Mayo Clinic College of Medicine,
Rochester, Minnesota

Sahil Khanna, MBBS
Senior Associate Consultant,
Division of Gastroenterology
    and Hepatology,
Mayo Clinic, Rochester, Minnesota;
Assistant Professor of Medicine,
Mayo Clinic College of Medicine,
Rochester, Minnesota

Daryl J. Kor, MD
Consultant,
Department of Anesthesiology,
Mayo Clinic, Rochester, Minnesota;
Associate Professor of Medicine,
Mayo Clinic College of Medicine,
Rochester, Minnesota

Christopher L. Kramer, MD
Fellow in Neurocritical Care Medicine,
Mayo School of Graduate
    Medical Education,
Mayo Clinic College of Medicine,
Rochester, Minnesota

Sarah J. Lee, MD, MPH
Fellow in Pulmonary
    and Critical Care Medicine,
Mayo School of Graduate
    Medical Education,
Mayo Clinic College of Medicine,
Rochester, Minnesota

Francis T. Lytle, MD
Consultant,
Division of Critical Care Medicine,
Department of Anesthesiology,
Mayo Clinic, Rochester, Minnesota;
Instructor in Anesthesiology,
Mayo Clinic College of Medicine,
Rochester, Minnesota

William J. Mauermann, MD
Consultant,
Department of Anesthesiology,
Mayo Clinic, Rochester, Minnesota;
Associate Professor of Anesthesiology,
Mayo Clinic College of Medicine,
Rochester, Minnesota

Teng Moua, MD
Senior Associate Consultant,
Division of Pulmonary
   and Critical Care Medicine,
Mayo Clinic, Rochester, Minnesota;
Assistant Professor of Medicine,
Mayo Clinic College of Medicine,
Rochester, Minnesota

Srikant Nannapaneni, MBBS
Fellow in Sleep Medicine,
Mayo School of Graduate Medical
   Education and Assistant
   Professor of Medicine,
Mayo Clinic College of Medicine,
Rochester, Minnesota

Sarah A. Narotzky, MD
Fellow in Pulmonary
   and Critical Care Medicine,
Mayo School of Graduate
   Medical Education,
Mayo Clinic College of Medicine,
Rochester, Minnesota

Sarah B. Nelson, PharmD, RPh
Pharmacist, Pharmacy Services,
Mayo Clinic, Rochester, Minnesota

Michael E. Nemergut, MD, PhD
Consultant,
Department of Anesthesiology,
Mayo Clinic, Rochester, Minnesota;
Assistant Professor of Anesthesiology
   and of Pediatrics,
Mayo Clinic College of Medicine,
Rochester, Minnesota

Matthew E. Nolan, MD
Resident in Internal Medicine,
Mayo School of Graduate
   Medical Education,
Mayo Clinic College of Medicine,
Rochester, Minnesota

John C. O'Horo, MD, MPH
Fellow in Infectious Diseases,
Mayo School of Graduate Medical
   Education and Assistant
   Professor of Medicine,
Mayo Clinic College of Medicine,
Rochester, Minnesota

James A. Onigkeit, MD
Consultant,
Department of Anesthesiology,
Mayo Clinic, Rochester, Minnesota;
Instructor in Anesthesiology,
Mayo Clinic College of Medicine,
Rochester, Minnesota

Jasleen R. Pannu, MBBS
Resident in Critical Care Medicine,
Mayo School of Graduate
    Medical Education,
Mayo Clinic College of Medicine,
Rochester, Minnesota

John G. Park, MD
Consultant, Division of Pulmonary
    and Critical Care Medicine,
Mayo Clinic, Rochester, Minnesota;
Assistant Professor of Medicine,
Mayo Clinic College of Medicine,
Rochester, Minnesota

Alejandro A. Rabinstein, MD
Consultant, Department of Neurology,
Mayo Clinic, Rochester, Minnesota;
Professor of Neurology,
Mayo Clinic College of Medicine,
Rochester, Minnesota

Misty A. Radosevich, MD
Resident in Anesthesiology,
Mayo School of Graduate
    Medical Education,
Mayo Clinic College of Medicine,
Rochester, Minnesota

Kannan Ramar, MBBS, MD
Consultant,
Division of Pulmonary and Critical
    Care Medicine,
Mayo Clinic, Rochester, Minnesota;
Associate Professor of Medicine,
Mayo Clinic College of Medicine,
Rochester, Minnesota

Dereddi Raja S. Reddy, MD
Fellow in Pulmonary and Critical
    Care Medicine,
Mayo School of Graduate Medical
    Education,
Mayo Clinic College of Medicine,
Rochester, Minnesota

Muhammad A. Rishi, MBBS
Fellow in Critical Care Medicine,
Mayo School of Graduate Medical
    Education and Assistant
    Professor of Medicine,
Mayo Clinic College of Medicine,
Rochester, Minnesota

Gregory J. Schears, MD
Consultant,
Department of Anesthesiology,
Mayo Clinic, Rochester, Minnesota;
Associate Professor of Anesthesiology,
Mayo Clinic College of Medicine,
Rochester, Minnesota

Hiroshi Sekiguchi, MD
Consultant,
Division of Pulmonary and Critical
    Care Medicine,
Mayo Clinic, Rochester, Minnesota;
Assistant Professor of Medicine,
Mayo Clinic College of Medicine,
Rochester, Minnesota

Bernardo J. Selim, MD
Consultant,
Division of Pulmonary and Critical
    Care Medicine,
Mayo Clinic, Rochester, Minnesota;
Assistant Professor of Medicine,
Mayo Clinic College of Medicine,
Rochester, Minnesota

Ronaldo A. Sevilla Berrios, MD
Fellow in Sleep Medicine,
Mayo School of Graduate Medical
    Education and Assistant
    Professor of Medicine,
Mayo Clinic College of Medicine,
Rochester, Minnesota

Shivani S. Shinde, MBBS
Fellow in Hematology and Oncology,
Mayo School of Graduate
    Medical Education,
Mayo Clinic College of Medicine,
Rochester, Minnesota

Raina Shivashankar, MD
Fellow in Gastroenterology
    and Hepatology,
Mayo School of Graduate
    Medical Education,
Mayo Clinic College of Medicine,
Rochester, Minnesota

Joseph H. Skalski, MD
Fellow in Critical Care Medicine,
Mayo School of Graduate Medical
    Education and Assistant
    Professor of Medicine,
Mayo Clinic College of Medicine,
Rochester, Minnesota

Nathan J. Smischney, MD
Senior Associate Consultant,
Division of Critical Care Medicine,
Mayo Clinic, Rochester, Minnesota;
Assistant Professor of Anesthesiology,
Mayo Clinic College of Medicine,
Rochester, Minnesota

Ulrich Specks, MD
Chair,
Division of Pulmonary
    and Critical Care Medicine,
Mayo Clinic, Rochester, Minnesota;
Professor of Medicine,
Mayo Clinic College of Medicine,
Rochester, Minnesota

Arun Subramanian, MBBS
Consultant,
Department of Anesthesiology,
Mayo Clinic, Rochester, Minnesota;
Assistant Professor of Anesthesiology,
Mayo Clinic College of Medicine,
Rochester, Minnesota

Shihab H. Sugeir, MD
Resident in Critical Care Medicine,
Mayo School of Graduate
    Medical Education,
Mayo Clinic College of Medicine,
Rochester, Minnesota

Rudy M. Tedja, DO
Fellow in Critical Care Medicine,
Mayo School of Graduate
    Medical Education,
Mayo Clinic College of Medicine,
Rochester, Minnesota

Lokendra Thakur, MBBS
Fellow in Pulmonary
    and Critical Care Medicine,
Mayo School of Graduate
    Medical Education,
Mayo Clinic College of Medicine,
Rochester, Minnesota

R. Thomas Tilbury, MD
Consultant,
Division of Cardiovascular Diseases,
Mayo Clinic, Rochester, Minnesota;
Assistant Professor,
Mayo Clinic College of Medicine,
Rochester, Minnesota

Sangita Trivedi, MBBS
Fellow in Pediatric
    Critical Care Medicine,
Mayo School of Graduate Medical
    Education and Assistant
    Professor of Pediatrics,
Mayo Clinic College of Medicine,
Rochester, Minnesota

Channing C. Twyner, MD
Resident in Anesthesiology,
Mayo School of Graduate
    Medical Education,
Mayo Clinic College of Medicine,
Rochester, Minnesota

Brendan T. Wanta, MD
Resident in Anesthesiology,
Mayo School of Graduate
    Medical Education,
Mayo Clinic College of Medicine,
Rochester, Minnesota

Blair Westerly, MD
Resident in Pulmonary
    and Critical Care Medicine,
Mayo School of Graduate
    Medical Education,
Mayo Clinic College of Medicine,
Rochester, Minnesota

Eelco F. M. Wijdicks, MD, PhD
Chair,
Division of Critical Care Neurology,
Mayo Clinic, Rochester, Minnesota;
Professor of Neurology,
Mayo Clinic College of Medicine,
Rochester, Minnesota

Amy W. Williams, MD
Consultant,
Division of Nephrology
  and Hypertension,
Mayo Clinic, Rochester, Minnesota;
Professor of Medicine,
Mayo Clinic College of Medicine,
Rochester, Minnesota

Erica D. Wittwer, MD, PhD
Fellow in Neurology,
Mayo School of Graduate
  Medical Education,
Mayo Clinic College of Medicine,
Rochester, Minnesota

Mark E. Wylam, MD
Consultant,
Division of Pulmonary and Critical
  Care Medicine,
Mayo Clinic, Rochester, Minnesota;
Associate Professor of Medicine,
Mayo Clinic College of Medicine,
Rochester, Minnesota

Section I

Cases

Dyspnea and Edema

BLAIR D. WESTERLY, MD,
AND HIROSHI SEKIGUCHI, MD

CASE PRESENTATION

A 58-year-old male smoker presented to a local emergency department with a 4-week history of progressive dyspnea. His symptoms included a productive cough with red-tinged sputum, orthopnea, and lower extremity edema. He recently spent nearly 2 consecutive days sitting in an automobile. Computed tomography showed segmental pulmonary emboli, right lower lobe consolidation, mediastinal lymphadenopathy, bilateral pleural effusion, and pericardial effusion. Bilevel positive pressure ventilation was begun, and he was transferred to the intensive care unit for further management. Upon transfer, vital signs included blood pressure, 98/78 mm Hg; heart rate, 110 beats per minute; respiratory rate, 40 breaths per minute; and oxygen saturation, 99% with 60% fraction of inspired oxygen (FIO_2). Physical examination showed elevated jugular venous pulse, rales in both lungs, decreased breath sounds in the right base, and tachycardia.

Bedside critical care ultrasonography showed a "swinging heart" with a large circumferential pericardial effusion, hyperdynamic left ventricle, diastolic collapse of the right atrium and ventricle, plethoric inferior vena cava, and a large right pleural effusion. With emergent ultrasonographically guided pericardiocentesis, 800 mL of hemorrhagic fluid was drained. Immediately after fluid removal, the patient's systolic blood pressure increased to 130 mm Hg with a concurrent decrease in heart rate to 80 to 90 beats per minute, confirming the diagnosis of cardiac tamponade. The patient subsequently underwent right thoracentesis, which drained 1,000 mL of hemorrhagic pleural fluid. Cytologic specimens from the pericardiocentesis and thoracentesis were positive for metastatic adenocarcinoma. The patient subsequently improved hemodynamically and was dismissed from the intensive care unit.

DISCUSSION

Successful management of obstructive shock requires early recognition and appropriate therapy targeted at the underlying physiology. Cardiac tamponade is a life-threatening obstructive shock caused by fluid accumulation in the pericardial sac, which compresses the cardiac chambers and inhibits normal filling. Dyspnea is the most common presenting symptom for patients with cardiac tamponade. The classic signs of soft heart sounds, elevated jugular venous pulse, and decreased blood pressure (Beck triad) were originally described when surgical patients had acute tamponade; however, they may be absent if fluid accumulation is slow (1). In a systematic review, pulsus paradoxus was reported to be the most sensitive examination finding in patients with cardiac tamponade (pooled sensitivity, 82%), followed by tachycardia (77%) and elevated jugular venous pulse (76%) (2). Conversely, sensitivity was only 26% for hypotension and 28% for diminished heart sounds (2). Pulsus paradoxus may be absent in the presence of other comorbid conditions, such as aortic regurgitation, positive pressure ventilation, increased left ventricular filling pressure, right ventricular hypertrophy, pulmonary hypertension, and local pericardial adhesions (2).

Cardiac critical care ultrasonography or critical care echocardiography is the noninvasive test of choice to evaluate pericardial effusion. Sonographic features suggestive of tamponade include inferior vena cava plethora and diastolic collapse of the right atrium and ventricle in the presence of pericardial effusion. *Inferior vena cava plethora*, defined as a decrease in diameter of less than 50% with inspiration, has been shown to have an overall sensitivity of 97%; however, it is only 40% specific (3). It represents the elevation in systemic venous pressure as pericardial pressure increases the intracardiac pressures. It can be absent in low-pressure tamponade related to trauma, dehydration, or surgery. Right atrial diastolic collapse is 55% sensitive and 88% specific; right ventricular diastolic collapse is 48% sensitive and 95% specific (3). Although they are relatively specific, regional tamponade and concurrent pulmonary hypertension may mask these findings (3). In research studies, various Doppler flow velocity recordings, such as an inspiratory reduction in mitral peak E-wave velocity by 30%, have been reported to be specific for the diagnosis (4). These Doppler measurements may further aid the diagnosis of tamponade; however, cardiac tamponade is a clinical diagnosis, and emergent pericardiocentesis should be considered even in the absence of classic echocardiographic findings. These situations include patients receiving mechanical ventilation and those who have regional tamponade with or without pulmonary hypertension (3,4).

Relief of hemodynamically significant pericardial effusion requires drainage of the fluid. Blind pericardiocentesis has been performed since the end of the 19th century; however, it carries considerable risk, such as puncture of thoracic or abdominal structures or even death, with reported mortality rates up to 6% (5). Use of echocardiography to guide needle placement has been shown to be safe and technically feasible (5). In the era of point-of-care ultrasonography, all pericardiocenteses should be performed under ultrasonographic guidance.

Cardiac tamponade is a clinical diagnosis suggested by symptoms, physical examination, and ultrasonographic findings, but it can be confirmed only by hemodynamic improvement with fluid removal. Critical care ultrasonography is helpful for identifying typical tamponade features; however, their absence does not rule out the presence of tamponade in patients receiving mechanical ventilation or in those with regional tamponade due to localized pericardial effusion or mass. Pericardiocentesis should be performed under ultrasonographic guidance.

REFERENCES

1. Guberman BA, Fowler NO, Engel PJ, Gueron M, Allen JM. Cardiac tamponade in medical patients. Circulation. 1981 Sep;64(3):633–40.
2. Roy CL, Minor MA, Brookhart MA, Choudhry NK. Does this patient with a pericardial effusion have cardiac tamponade? JAMA. 2007 Apr 25;297(16):1810–8.
3. Himelman RB, Kircher B, Rockey DC, Schiller NB. Inferior vena cava plethora with blunted respiratory response: a sensitive echocardiographic sign of cardiac tamponade. J Am Coll Cardiol. 1988 Dec;12(6):1470–7.

4. Klein AL, Abbara S, Agler DA, Appleton CP, Asher CR, Hoit B, et al. American Society of Echocardiography clinical recommendations for multimodality cardiovascular imaging of patients with pericardial disease: endorsed by the Society for Cardiovascular Magnetic Resonance and Society of Cardiovascular Computed Tomography. J Am Soc Echocardiogr. 2013 Sep;26(9):965–1012.e15.

5. Tsang TS, Freeman WK, Sinak LJ, Seward JB. Echocardiographically guided pericardiocentesis: evolution and state-of-the-art technique. Mayo Clin Proc. 1998 Jul;73(7):647–52.

An Electrical Problem

RONALDO A. SEVILLA BERRIOS, MD, AND ERICA D. WITTWER, MD, PhD

CASE PRESENTATION

A 50-year-old man with type 2 diabetes mellitus and paroxysmal atrial tachycardia presented with a 1-week history of intermittent chest pain. An initial electrocardiogram showed ST-segment depression on the inferior leads (II, III, and aVF) and ST-segment elevation of 2 to 3 mm in the lateral leads (V_3 through V_6). In the emergency department, he was treated with aspirin, nitroglycerin, metoprolol, clopidogrel, and a heparin bolus. An emergent coronary angiogram showed a critical left main coronary artery lesion that required emergent coronary artery bypass surgery. The patient's postoperative course was complicated by refractory cardiogenic shock requiring extracorporeal membrane oxygenation (ECMO) and intra-aortic balloon pump support.

Later that day in the intensive care unit, refractory ventricular tachycardia (VT) developed in the patient. He was defibrillated and dosed with several antiarrhythmics, including amiodarone, lidocaine, procainamide, magnesium, esmolol, and calcium, over a 2-hour period. Ultimately, the VT episode terminated with overdrive pacing of epicardial pacing leads placed at the time of surgery. Although this episode was quite prolonged and the patient received over 20 defibrillations, his organ perfusion was maintained with ECMO support without significant systemic hypoperfusion. However, his cardiac function diminished, and he required multiple inotropic agents and vasopressors and prolonged ECMO support.

The patient was deemed not to be a cardiac transplant candidate, and he refused implantation of ventricular assist devices or prolonged life support through artificial means. He transitioned to comfort measures only and died.

DISCUSSION

Since the mid 2000s, cardiovascular disease has been the leading cause of death among Americans (1). A large proportion of that mortality is from fatal arrhythmias. In the Thrombolysis in Myocardial Infarction (TIMI) II trial, 2% of patients had sustained, life-threatening arrhythmias in the first 24 hours after an intervention and had a significantly higher in-hospital mortality than the other 98% without sustained, life-threatening arrhythmias (20.4% vs 1.6%) (2).

Arrhythmias are an important complication of acute coronary syndromes and can be clinically challenging to manage. *Sustained VT* and *ventricular fibrillation* (VF) are the most frequent hemodynamically relevant arrhythmias and are defined as ventricular arrhythmias lasting more than 30 seconds and requiring an intervention for termination (3). The Assessment of Pexelizumab in Acute Myocardial Infarction (APEX AMI) trial data were used to evaluate the prognosis of 329 patients who had ST-elevation myocardial infarction and episodes of sustained VT or VF. In this study, 90-day mortality was significantly greater among those with sustained ventricular arrhythmia compared to those without (23.2% vs 3.6%). Outcomes were also significantly worse for patients with arrhythmias arising after catheterization compared to before catheterization (33.3% vs 17.2%) (4).

The cornerstone of treatment of ventricular arrhythmia is early electrical cardioversion or defibrillation with adjuvant suppressant pharmacology therapy as outlined by the American Heart Association Advanced Cardiovascular Life Support guidelines. When this strategy fails, *electrical storm* can develop, defined as a cluster of 3 or more episodes of VT or VF that occur within 24 hours and require defibrillation. These could be perpetuated by other triggers, such as electrolyte abnormalities, enhanced sympathetic tone, and genetic abnormalities (eg, Brugada syndrome, long QT syndrome, or early repolarization syndrome). Most often, electrical storm is multifactorial and sustained control is a challenge.

With the complex underlying physiopathology of VT or VF, refractory cases require the use of combination therapy. Pharmacologic treatment includes sympathetic blockade (selective β-antagonist, direct left stellate ganglion blockage, and propofol) and antiarrhythmics with synergistic effects (class IB antiarrhythmics, such as lidocaine, and class III antiarrhythmics, such as amiodarone). Nonpharmacologic therapy includes overdrive pacing and supportive measures such as ECMO and intra-aortic balloon pump in hemodynamically unstable patients. Ablation can be used in hemodynamically stable patients. The most effective approach is to correct the underlying cause in combination with pharmacologic and nonpharmacologic means (5).

REFERENCES

1. Murphy SL, Xu J, Kochanek KD. Deaths: preliminary data for 2010. National vital statistics reports; vol 60 no 4. Hyattsville (MD): National Center for Health Statistics; 2012.

2. Berger PB, Ruocco NA, Ryan TJ, Frederick MM, Podrid PJ. Incidence and significance of ventricular tachycardia and fibrillation in the absence of hypotension or heart failure in acute myocardial infarction treated with recombinant tissue-type plasminogen activator: results from the Thrombolysis in Myocardial Infarction (TIMI) Phase II trial. J Am Coll Cardiol. 1993 Dec;22(7):1773–9.

3. Eifling M, Razavi M, Massumi A. The evaluation and management of electrical storm. Tex Heart Inst J. 2011;38(2):111–21.

4. Mehta RH, Starr AZ, Lopes RD, Hochman JS, Widimsky P, Pieper KS, et al; APEX AMI Investigators. Incidence of and outcomes associated with ventricular tachycardia or fibrillation in patients undergoing primary percutaneous coronary intervention. JAMA. 2009 May 6;301(17):1779–89.

5. Hsieh J-C, Bui M, Yallapragda S, Huang SKS. Current management of electrical storm. Acta Cardiol Sin. 2011;27:71–6.

Hypertension

SRIKANT NANNAPANENI, MBBS, LISBETH Y. GARCIA ARGUELLO, MD, AND JOHN G. PARK, MD

CASE PRESENTATION

A 66-year-old white man with a medical history of atrial fibrillation, hypertension treated with atenolol and lisinopril, and obstructive sleep apnea managed with continuous positive airway pressure was hospitalized for labile blood pressures. On the day of hospitalization, he underwent outpatient bone spur surgery on his right foot; after the procedure, bradycardia developed and was initially treated with intravenous fluids and glycopyrrolate. Subsequently, a hypertensive crisis developed, resulting in pulmonary edema, which was initially managed with intravenous furosemide and a nitroprusside drip. However, the patient became hemodynamically unstable, requiring intubation and initiation of multiple antihypertensive drugs, including nicardipine, atenolol, lisinopril, and labetalol. Computed tomography (CT) of the chest showed a 5-cm soft tissue mass; magnetic resonance imaging (MRI) showed a 7.1×4.2×5.0-cm mass in the retroperitoneal and left para-aortic areas with extension to the proximal celiac and superior mesenteric arteries. An electrocardiogram showed a non–ST elevation myocardial infarction; troponin levels were elevated. Coronary angiography showed normal coronary arteries; ejection fraction was reduced (40%). Catecholamine levels were elevated: dopamine 41 pg/mL, epinephrine 296 pg/mL, and norepinephrine 1,743 pg/mL.

By the third day of hospitalization, the patient's blood pressure was well controlled with phenoxybenzamine, amlodipine, and phentolamine. Transthoracic echocardiography showed moderate left ventricular enlargement and an ejection fraction of 71%. A metaiodobenzylguanidine (MIBG) scan, recommended by an endocrinologist and a general surgeon, confirmed the diagnosis of para-aortic paraganglioma without metastasis.

The patient was discharged home with his blood pressure continuing to improve with phenoxybenzamine and atenolol. In a subsequent operation, the catecholamine-secreting paraganglioma was successfully removed, and he had a good clinical recovery.

DISCUSSION

Pheochromocytomas are rare catecholamine-secreting tumors that arise from the chromaffin cells in the adrenal medulla and from the sympathetic ganglia (also called paragangliomas) outside the adrenal. The annual incidence is less than 1 per 100,000 persons. Although the classic textbook presentation is the triad of episodic headache, sweating, and tachycardia, the clinical presentation can range from an incidental discovery of an adrenal mass on imaging studies in an asymptomatic patient to hypertensive crises resulting in acute end-organ complications. The key to diagnosis is to have a high degree of clinical awareness. For a confirmed pheochromocytoma, early and aggressive therapy with a combination of α- and β-adrenergic blockers results in effective blood pressure control before definitive management (ie, surgery) can be considered.

Neuroendocrine tumors (NETs) cover a spectrum of malignancies derived from a common cell line and unified by the presence of neuroendocrine cells (1). The annual incidence of NET is 5.25 per 100,000 persons (2). Despite this low incidence, the prevalence has increased 5-fold since the 1980s (2). The incidence is equal between both sexes but is higher among whites. The main risk factors for NET are genetic factors and a long history of diabetes mellitus, especially for patients with gastric NETs (3).

NETs may develop at any location, but the most common sites are the gastrointestinal tract (67%) and lungs (27%) (2,4). NETs are classified in various ways, including adrenal location: In this classification, the most common are intra-adrenal (pheochromocytoma; 80%-85%) and extra-adrenal (sympathetic and parasympathetic paraganglioma; 15%-20%) (5).

Most patients with NETs are asymptomatic, and the tumors are found incidentally. However, the symptoms vary depending on tumor location (3). NETs located in the adrenal gland produce catecholamines; the symptoms depend on the amount of catecholamines excreted. Thus, the main signs and symptoms include intermittent hypertension, palpitations, headache, sweating, and pallor (5).

The diagnosis of pheochromocytoma and paraganglioma is based on measurement of fractional metanephrines in a 24-hour urine sample or plasma (5). If patients have paroxysmal symptoms, the sample should preferably be collected shortly after the paroxysm. Plasma tests for metanephrines and catecholamines have a higher sensitivity and result in more false-positive results. When plasma samples are collected, the patient should be in a supine position to decrease the chance of false-positive results (5). CT or MRI of the abdomen is indicated to localize the tumor. MIBG imaging is useful for diagnosing metastatic disease (1).

After a diagnosis of pheochromocytoma is confirmed, surgical resection is the definitive therapy for local and regional disease (5). Patients can have chronic volume contraction from adrenergic overactivity, and preoperative volume expansion is recommended to reduce postoperative hypotension. Also, to minimize the complication of a catecholamine surge intraoperatively, patients should be treated medically for at least 10 to 14 days preoperatively (1). The number of complications during surgery has been shown to decrease to less than 3% with α-blockade (1,5). A β-blocker should be added to prevent tachyarrhythmias and angina (5).

Pheochromocytomas are rare but clinically important tumors of neuroendocrine origin associated with clinical symptoms mediated by excessive production of catecholamines. The clinical presentation can range from asymptomatic to the classic triad of paroxysmal symptoms to malignant hypertension. Diagnosis is based on quantification of catecholamines (the gold standard) followed by imaging studies (CT scan to localize the tumor followed by MIBG scan for confirmation). Combined α- and β-blocker therapy usually results in effective blood pressure control. The use of β-blockers alone can elevate the blood pressure (and cause clinical worsening) because of the unopposed α-adrenergic effects of elevated catecholamines. Adequate blood pressure control is essential before surgical resection of the tumor.

REFERENCES

1. Vinik AI, Woltering EA, Warner RR, Caplin M, O'Dorisio TM, Wiseman GA, et al; North American Neuroendocrine Tumor Society (NANETS). NANETS consensus guidelines for the diagnosis of neuroendocrine tumor. Pancreas. 2010 Aug;39(6):713–34.

2. Yao JC, Hassan M, Phan A, Dagohoy C, Leary C, Mares JE, et al. One hundred years after "carcinoid": epidemiology of and prognostic factors for neuroendocrine tumors in 35,825 cases in the United States. J Clin Oncol. 2008 Jun 20;26(18):3063–72.

3. Hassan MM, Phan A, Li D, Dagohoy CG, Leary C, Yao JC. Risk factors associated with neuroendocrine tumors: a U.S.-based case-control study. Int J Cancer. 2008 Aug 15;123(4):867–73.

4. Taal BG, Visser O. Epidemiology of neuroendocrine tumours. Neuroendocrinology. 2004;80 Suppl 1:3–7.

5. Chen H, Sippel RS, O'Dorisio MS, Vinik AI, Lloyd RV, Pacak K; North American Neuroendocrine Tumor Society (NANETS). The North American Neuroendocrine Tumor Society consensus guideline for the diagnosis and management of neuroendocrine tumors: pheochromocytoma, paraganglioma, and medullary thyroid cancer. Pancreas. 2010 Aug;39(6):775–83.

A Rare Cause of Liver Failure

ALICE GALLO DE MORAES, MD,
SARAH A. NAROTZKY, MD,
AND TENG MOUA, MD

CASE PRESENTATION

A 56-year-old nonsmoker was initially admitted to a local hospital for new-onset jaundice and hypotension. He had an elevated international normalized ratio and bilirubin level and an acute-on-chronic kidney injury. Abdominal ultrasonography and computed tomography of the abdomen and pelvis showed no hepatomegaly, ascites, or biliary dilatation. Results for hepatitis viral serologies, antinuclear antibody, human immunodeficiency virus antibody, and anti–smooth muscle antibody were also negative. His total bilirubin level increased to 22.0 mg/dL, and he was transferred with a diagnosis of subacute liver failure and plans for possible liver biopsy.

Other pertinent history included recent-onset atrial fibrillation, morbid obesity, and obstructive sleep apnea. The atrial fibrillation was symptomatic and difficult to treat; multiple rate-controlling agents, including sotalol and dronedarone, were ineffective. Ultimately, amiodarone was started 3 days before admission.

Given the negative imaging and laboratory findings, the patient's liver failure was considered a possible drug-induced result of the recent initiation of amiodarone. However, the patient's liver function worsened despite discontinuation of the drug. Additionally, medical records from another facility showed that total bilirubin was elevated several weeks before amiodarone use, so this agent was less likely to have caused subacute liver failure.

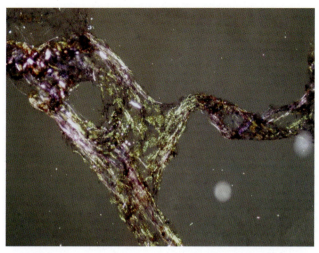

FIGURE 4.1. Fat Pad Aspirate. The apple-green birefringence on polarized light microscopy is consistent with amyloid.

Echocardiography showed normal ejection fraction, moderately increased left ventricular thickness (19 mm), and mild right ventricular dysfunction. The findings were reported as "consistent with an underlying infiltrative process." Given the patient's ongoing coagulopathy and hemodynamic instability, the risk of complication with liver biopsy was unacceptably high; fat pad aspiration was performed instead (Figure 4.1). Histopathologic findings were consistent with AL amyloid; the elevated λ and κ free light chain values were 53.9 mg/dL and 6.24 mg/dL, respectively. Given the advanced disease and limited treatment options, the patient was discharged home with hospice care after discussion with palliative care, oncology, and critical care specialists.

DISCUSSION

Amyloidosis is a rare, progressive, and often fatal disease that is notably difficult to diagnose because of nonspecific serologic and imaging studies during the initial stages. However, early recognition and diagnosis are crucial for treatment, which may limit and reverse organ dysfunction. The exact incidence of amyloidosis is unknown. In the United States, systemic light chain–related amyloidosis (ie, AL amyloidosis) has an incidence of 5.1 to 12.8 cases per million person-years (1); it occurs in all geographic locations and affects all races, with a mean age at diagnosis of 65 years.

AL amyloidosis is a clonal, nonproliferative disorder in which plasma cells produce a monoclonal light chain protein of the κ or λ type. The light chain proteins misfold and form β-pleated sheets, which are insoluble and deposit in tissues. The β-pleated sheet configuration is responsible for the Congo red–positive staining when viewed under polarized light (2).

The initial workup includes serum and urine protein electrophoresis if amyloidosis is suspected. If those results are negative, the diagnosis of amyloidosis is unlikely. If they are positive, fat pad and bone marrow biopsy specimens should be obtained and stained with Congo red. A positive bone marrow biopsy associated with positive fat pad findings may identify only 85% of patients. Hence, when biopsy findings are negative but suspicion is high for AL amyloidosis, biopsy of a suspected clinically involved organ may be necessary.

Amyloidosis may affect any organ, although it generally spares the central nervous system. The heart and kidneys are most commonly affected by infiltrated insoluble fibrils. Half of presenting patients have some form of hepatic deposition; however, the liver is rarely the dominant organ affected at presentation (3).

Lethargy and abdominal pain are the most common presenting symptoms in patients with hepatic involvement. Massive hepatomegaly is nearly always present. Gastrointestinal tract involvement is common but usually asymptomatic. Occult bleeding, malabsorption, perforation, and intestinal obstruction may occur. Macroglossia, which is highly suggestive of AL amyloidosis, is recognized in only 15% of cases (4).

Patients with hepatic amyloidosis present primarily with a cholestatic clinical picture, with elevated bilirubin levels (median, 15.2 mg/dL) and alkaline phosphatase levels (median, 1,132 U/L) (3). Bilirubin is predominantly direct in most patients, with transaminase levels usually normal or mildly elevated. The pathogenesis of cholestasis in hepatic amyloidosis is unknown. Common findings on liver biopsy include severe infiltration of the liver parenchyma, leading to increased sinusoidal pressure, with resultant hepatocyte atrophy. Thrombocytosis is often associated with amyloid-related severe intrahepatic cholestasis and is thought to be a consequence of functional hyposplenism (3). Rarely, a severe form of cholestatic hepatitis may occur, which is usually rapidly fatal (4).

The treatment of liver failure often requires intensive care that is directed toward supportive therapy and treatment of underlying causes. If encephalopathy develops, early intubation is recommended for airway protection. Coagulation factor abnormalities should be corrected if bleeding is present or if procedures are planned. Cardiovascular support should focus on early restoration of circulatory volume and oxygen-carrying capacity. If a vasopressor is needed, norepinephrine is preferred with or without adjunctive use of vasopressin (5).

Amyloidosis-specific treatment relies on chemotherapy aimed at suppressing plasma cell clones secreting amyloid-forming light chains. The combination of an alkylating agent with high-dose dexamethasone has proved effective in about two-thirds of patients, with median survival of 5.1 years after treatment (4).

Stem cell transplant may be an option for eliminating amyloidogenic light chains produced by the clonal plasma cell population. Its biggest limitation is availability: Less than 20% to 25% of patients are eligible, with a 10-year survival of 43% (2). Survival depends on the hematologic response to therapy and the extent of disease at diagnosis.

REFERENCES

1. Falk RH, Comenzo RL, Skinner M. The systemic amyloidoses. N Engl J Med. 1997 Sep 25;337(13):898–909.
2. Gertz MA. Immunoglobulin light chain amyloidosis: 2013 update on diagnosis, prognosis, and treatment. Am J Hematol. 2013 May;88(5):416–25.
3. Hydes TJ, Aspinall RJ. Subacute liver failure secondary to amyloid light-chain amyloidosis. Gastroenterol Hepatol (NY). 2012 Mar;8(3):205–8.
4. Desport E, Bridoux F, Sirac C, Delbes S, Bender S, Fernandez B, et al; Centre national de référence pour l'amylose AL et les autres maladies par dépôts d'immunoglobulines monoclonales. Al amyloidosis. Orphanet J Rare Dis. 2012 Aug 21;7:54.
5. Eefsen M, Dethloff T, Frederiksen HJ, Hauerberg J, Hansen BA, Larsen FS. Comparison of terlipressin and noradrenalin on cerebral perfusion, intracranial pressure and cerebral extra-cellular concentrations of lactate and pyruvate in patients with acute liver failure in need of inotropic support. J Hepatol. 2007 Sep;47(3):381–6. Epub 2007 May 30.

Shortness of Breath

CARLOS J. RACEDO AFRICANO, MD, AND DARLENE R. NELSON, MD

CASE PRESENTATION

A previously healthy 32-year-old man, originally from South Asia and now a university student in the Midwest, was admitted to the medical intensive care unit for hypoxemic respiratory failure and septic shock. He had no known past medical or surgical history, no significant family history or personal history of substance abuse, and no known risk factor for human immunodeficiency virus (HIV) infection.

A few months before presentation, cough and fever developed and persisted. The patient was evaluated at the university student health clinic and received several courses of antibiotics, including azithromycin, ceftriaxone, and cefdinir without clear improvement in his symptoms. He was eventually referred to a local pulmonologist 10 days before presentation; a chest radiograph showed lower lobe consolidation with pleural effusion. The patient was admitted to a local hospital for further management and workup.

His vital signs were remarkable for a blood pressure of 80/50 mm Hg and a heart rate of 126 beats per minute. He was in severe respiratory distress and diaphoretic, with decreased breath sounds at the left base and rhonchi in the rest of the left hemithorax. Physical examination findings were otherwise unremarkable. Laboratory results included a leukocyte count of 17×10^9/L with neutrophilia, a lactate level of 2.1 mmol/L, and acute renal failure with metabolic acidosis. The patient received intravenous fluids, broad-spectrum antibiotics (cefepime, vancomycin, and doxycycline), and norepinephrine. Progressive hypoxemic respiratory failure developed, and he underwent emergent intubation. At that time, the leukocyte count had increased to 30×10^9/L. A new chest radiograph showed bilateral alveolar infiltrates and a large left-sided pleural effusion (Figure 5.1). Results were negative for blood and respiratory cultures (sputum), multiple viral serologies (including HIV), and testing for *Legionella, Mycoplasma,* and *Streptococcus pneumoniae.* Bronchoalveolar lavage showed many neutrophils and fungal elements, which increased suspicion for *Blastomyces,* and was negative for *Pneumocystis.* The patient was given amphotericin B lipid complex (5 mg/kg). Thoracentesis showed a pH of 7.1 and a leukocyte count of 2.5×10^9/L, consistent with complicated parapneumonic effusion. His respiratory status decreased further (ratio of Pao_2 to fraction of inspired oxygen [Fio_2], 82). He eventually became anuric and required renal replacement therapy. Because of his worsening clinical status, the patient was transferred to our institution for further evaluation and treatment.

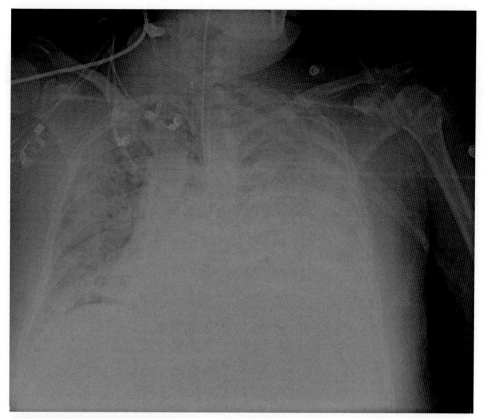

FIGURE 5.1. Chest Radiograph. The radiograph shows bilateral infiltrates with left-sided pleural effusion.

The patient arrived intubated. His F_{IO_2} was 1.0, positive end-expiratory pressure was 10 cm H_2O, and minute ventilation was 11.7 L/min. He was receiving norepinephrine 0.05 mcg/kg per minute for pressure support, he was febrile (39°C), and his oxygen saturation by pulse oximetry was 91%. His leukocyte count was 61×10^9/L (72% neutrophils, 3% lymphocytes, and 1% monocytes). Echocardiography showed a hyperdynamic ventricle but was otherwise normal. A 32F chest tube was placed to drain the complicated pleural effusion. A second bronchoalveolar lavage again showed *Blastomyces dermatitidis*, and treatment with amphotericin B was continued, with the addition of methylprednisolone 60 mg intravenously every 6 hours, because the use of intravenous corticosteroids has been reported in the treatment of acute respiratory distress syndrome (ARDS) caused by blastomycosis (1).

The patient recovered from respiratory failure after a prolonged stay in the intensive care unit. He was discharged to a rehabilitation facility without any oxygen requirement, but he continued to require hemodialysis.

DISCUSSION

Blastomycosis is a multisystem disease with a predilection for respiratory and cutaneous involvement caused by the dimorphic fungus *Blastomyces dermatitidis*. In North America, the organism is most commonly found in the Midwest and in parts of Canada and Mexico. Worldwide, the majority of cases are reported in northern India (1). Most cases of blastomycosis occur in males; although the incidence appears to be higher in African Americans, socioeconomic factors seem to be more important than race. The disease equally attacks immunocompetent and immunocompromised hosts, including those with HIV infection, and only infrequently occurs as an opportunistic infection (2,3). However, evidence clearly shows that early dissemination, ARDS, and increased mortality are more frequent among AIDS patients.

Primary infection is most often caused by inhalation of conidia or by contamination through skin trauma. Virtually all patients have pulmonary involvement that ranges from acute pneumonia and resolution without dissemination to pneumonia with multiorgan involvement or severe pulmonary disease with ARDS. Although ARDS occurs in less than 10% of patients, when it is present, the estimated mortality rate is 50% to 89% in spite of adequate therapy (2).

Extrapulmonary disease may involve (in decreasing order of frequency) the skin, bone, genitourinary organs, reticuloendothelial system, and gastrointestinal tract.

The diagnosis is made by culture and microscopic demonstration of the yeast. Serology has good sensitivity (about 80%), but specificity is poor and cross-reactions with *Histoplasma* are possible. Antigen detection in urine (with polymerase chain reaction [PCR]) has similar sensitivity (83%-90%), but cross reactions occur with other fungi (3). PCR is fast but expensive and is currently used mainly in research (3).

Treatment is based on the severity of the disease. Although the definition of *mild* and *severe* varies, mild disease is managed with itraconazole 200 mg orally twice daily for 6 to 12 months. Life-threatening disease typically requires treatment with amphotericin B deoxycholate (0.7-1.0 mg/kg daily) or amphotericin B lipid complex for patients with renal failure (5 mg/kg daily). Either medication is continued until the patient shows clinical improvement, and then itraconazole is given. If ARDS is present, the use of systemic corticosteroids ($\geq$40-60 mg prednisone daily) for 2 weeks should be considered (2,3). Immunocompromised hosts are treated as having severe disease, and itraconazole therapy is maintained until immunity recovers or for lifetime suppression if the immunosuppressed state is permanent.

Blastomycosis can be a severe life-threatening disease and should be considered in patients living in endemic areas if they have a pulmonary infection that is unresponsive to conventional therapy.

REFERENCES

1. Lopez-Martinez R, Mendez-Tovar LJ. Blastomycosis. Clin Dermatol. 2012 Nov-Dec;30(6): 565–72.

2. Lahm T, Neese S, Thornburg AT, Ober MD, Sarosi GA, Hage CA. Corticosteroids for blastomycosis-induced ARDS: a report of two patients and review of the literature. Chest. 2008 Jun;133(6):1478–80.

3. Limper AH, Knox KS, Sarosi GA, Ampel NM, Bennett JE, Catanzaro A, et al; American Thoracic Society Fungal Working Group. An official American Thoracic Society statement: treatment of fungal infections in adult pulmonary and critical care patients. Am J Respir Crit Care Med. 2011 Jan 1;183(1):96–128.

Acute Respiratory Failure in a Young Smoker

MAZEN O. AL-QADI, MBBS, AND BERNARDO J. SELIM, MD

CASE PRESENTATION

A 26-year-old man who was an active smoker with a history of mild childhood asthma was transferred from another hospital for management of acute respiratory failure. He was in his usual state of health until the week before his illness, when fever, dry cough, dyspnea, pleuritic chest pain, and malaise developed. As an outpatient, he was prescribed antibiotics for presumed community-acquired pneumonia. However, his symptoms progressed, and within 5 days bilateral pulmonary infiltrates with pleural effusion developed, leading to respiratory failure that required mechanical ventilation. The week before the onset of symptoms, the patient was exposed to dust and bird droppings while cutting down trees.

When he arrived in the intensive care unit, the patient was hemodynamically stable and was receiving mechanical ventilation. Therapy for infectious agents was expanded to include coverage for regional fungal organisms, such as *Histoplasma*, with the addition of amphotericin B. Bronchoscopy was performed, and bronchoalveolar lavage (BAL) fluid was evaluated for a differential blood count and microbiology evaluation. BAL showed marked eosinophilia (32%) with no evidence of diffuse alveolar hemorrhage. Bacterial, viral, and fungal cultures were negative. Therapy was started with methylprednisolone 125 mg intravenously daily for 2 days, with a dramatic resolution of lung infiltrates. The patient was extubated within 48 hours and discharged home with oral prednisone 60 mg daily to be tapered over 4 weeks.

DISCUSSION

Acute respiratory failure is a common reason for intensive care unit admission, and it is associated with high mortality among patients with multiorgan failure. In healthy immunocompetent adults, acute respiratory failure may develop from various causes, including acute respiratory distress syndrome (ARDS). ARDS is characterized by acute onset of severe hypoxemia and bilateral pulmonary infiltrates due to noncardiogenic pulmonary edema. However, young adults may have acute hypoxemic respiratory failure with diffuse, noninfectious infiltrations and pathophysiologic features and outcomes that are different from ARDS. Therefore, the following conditions should be considered in the differential diagnosis:

- Cardiogenic pulmonary edema (eg, viral myocarditis)
- Acute organizing pneumonia
- Acute eosinophilic pneumonia (AEP)
- Acute hypersensitivity pneumonitis
- Diffuse alveolar hemorrhage (DAH)
- Acute interstitial pneumonia

Except in cases of cardiogenic pulmonary edema, bronchoscopy with BAL is usually performed to obtain samples for microbiology testing, as well as for cell type and differential blood count (eg, eosinophilia for AEP and hemosiderin-laden alveolar macrophages for DAH).

AEP is a rare disorder characterized by severe respiratory failure (commonly requiring mechanical ventilation), bilateral lung infiltrates, and pulmonary eosinophilia. The condition is frequently misdiagnosed as ARDS because of the acute onset of illness (typically <1 week), severe hypoxemia, and findings on chest imaging. The disease occurs mostly in young adults (20-35 years old) and more commonly in males. Most patients have a history of recent exposure to an environmental or occupational stimulus (eg, heavy dust), with tobacco smoke being the most common (1), and in many patients, AEP develops when the patient resumes smoking after a period of abstinence. Patients with AEP present with nonspecific symptoms, including dry cough, dyspnea, chest pain, fever, and fatigue. Respiratory failure rapidly ensues within a few days. Extrapulmonary organ failure is unusual and may point to an alternative diagnosis (eg, Churg-Strauss vasculitis with DAH).

Laboratory test results are usually nonspecific, and the peripheral eosinophil count is usually normal at presentation, but eosinophilia may develop as the disease progresses (2). An elevated eosinophil count (usually >25%) on BAL is a prominent finding. The serum immunoglobulin E level may be elevated (3). Radiographic features of AEP include diffuse bilateral air space consolidation with reticular abnormalities resembling pulmonary edema. Bilateral pleural effusion is a common finding, with an elevated eosinophil count in the fluid.

The diagnosis of AEP is based on a consistent history (recent environmental exposure), radiographic findings, and elevated eosinophils on BAL (after exclusion of other conditions, such as infections or DAH). The following criteria are proposed for diagnosing AEP (3):

- Acute illness (usually <5-7 days)
- Diffuse bilateral pulmonary infiltrates on chest imaging
- PaO_2 <60 mm Hg or oxygen saturation <90%
- Elevated eosinophils (>25%) on BAL, or prominent eosinophilic infiltrate on lung biopsy
- Exclusion of pulmonary infection and other causes of pulmonary infiltrates with eosinophilia

Therapy includes use of broad-spectrum antibiotics appropriate for severe community-acquired pneumonia until infection is excluded. Most patients require ventilator support for severe hypoxic respiratory failure. Systemic corticosteroid therapy is effective, and most patients show considerable improvement in oxygenation within a few days, so that mechanical ventilation is no longer required. The optimal dose and duration of corticosteroid therapy is not well studied. Methylprednisolone 60 to 125 mg intravenously every 6 hours (or prednisone 40-60 mg orally if the patient can take oral medication) for 1 to 3 days has been used, with the dose tapered over 2 to 4 weeks (4). A dramatic response to corticosteroids usually supports the diagnosis, and failure of therapy should raise concern about an alternative pathologic process.

REFERENCES

1. Philit F, Etienne-Mastroianni B, Parrot A, Guerin C, Robert D, Cordier JF. Idiopathic acute eosinophilic pneumonia: a study of 22 patients. Am J Respir Crit Care Med. 2002 Nov 1;166(9):1235–9.

2. Allen JN, Davis WB. Eosinophilic lung diseases. Am J Respir Crit Care Med. 1994 Nov;150(5 Pt 1):1423–38.

3. Hayakawa H, Sato A, Toyoshima M, Imokawa S, Taniguchi M. A clinical study of idiopathic eosinophilic pneumonia. Chest. 1994 May;105(5):1462–6.

4. Rhee CK, Min KH, Yim NY, Lee JE, Lee NR, Chung MP, et al. Clinical characteristics and corticosteroid treatment of acute eosinophilic pneumonia. Eur Respir J. 2013 Feb;41(2):402–9. Epub 2012 May 17.

Shock

MAZEN O. AL-QADI, MBBS, JOHN C. O'HORO, MD, MPH, AND LARRY M. BADDOUR, MD

CASE PRESENTATION

A 60-year-old man presented to the emergency department with fever (40°C) and change in mental status. His wife mentioned that on the day before presentation he was nauseated and vomiting, which was initially attributed to gastroenteritis. He had surgery for acute cholecystitis 4 weeks before this presentation, and his postoperative course was complicated by purulent drainage from the surgical site. Upon arrival at the emergency department, he had a toxic appearance; his blood pressure was 90/60 mm Hg, his heart rate was 140 beats per minute, and his respiratory rate was 38 breaths per minute. In addition, he had diffuse macular erythema of the trunk and extremities but normal mucous membranes.

Initial laboratory tests showed leukocytosis (white blood cells 26×10^9/L), thrombocytopenia (platelets 97×10^9/L; platelets decreased further to 34×10^9/L within 48 hours after admission), acute kidney injury (serum creatinine 5.3 mg/dL), elevated lactate (12.5 mmol/L), and normal liver function test results. Deep swab culture of the abdominal wound grew *Staphylococcus aureus*.

The diagnosis of probable toxic shock syndrome (TSS) was made from the clinical presentation (shock with multiorgan failure and erythroderma) and the positive wound culture. The illness was aggressively managed with early goal-directed therapy with intravenous fluid resuscitation, vasopressors, broad-spectrum antibiotics (piperacillin-tazobactam, ciprofloxacin, and vancomycin), and débridement of the abdominal wound. The patient also required renal replacement therapy. The antibiotics were de-escalated to piperacillin-tazobactam on day 5. His condition improved, and he was transferred from the intensive care unit after 10 days.

DISCUSSION

TSS is a severe, toxin-mediated illness that results from dysregulation of the host inflammatory response and is characterized by hypotension with multiorgan dysfunction. Although TSS was originally described as occurring in menstruating women, in more recent surveys 50% of cases occur in men and nonmenstruating women.

The disease is caused by toxin-producing strains of *S aureus* (including methicillin-resistant *S aureus*), group A streptococci (GAS) (also known as *Streptococcus pyogenes*), and other β-hemolytic streptococci, although it can be caused by other bacteria (eg, *Clostridium* species, the viridans streptococci group, and coagulase-negative staphylococci), albeit very rarely. These bacteria produce superantigens that directly unleash inflammatory cells, bypassing the usual interaction with antigen-presenting cells, and stimulate polyclonal T-cell activation, resulting in massive cytokine release. Typical antigens are processed by antigen-presenting cells bound to class II major histocompatibility complex molecules, allowing specific clonal activation of an appropriate T-cell line. Superantigens nonspecifically bind to class II major histocompatibility complex molecules, causing polyclonal activation of up to 20% of T-cell lines and a resultant "cytokine storm," which is responsible for the classic presentation of TSS (1).

Clinically, patients with TSS usually present with fever, severe myalgia, skin rash or diffuse erythema, hypotension, and multiorgan dysfunction. In addition, patients may have nonspecific symptoms, such as nausea, vomiting, headache, or change in mental status. Desquamation of the skin (typically of the palms and soles) may occur in a later stage of the syndrome. Box 7.1 summarizes the diagnostic criteria for TSS (2,3).

BOX 7.1.
DIAGNOSTIC CRITERIA FOR TSS

Streptococcal TSS[a]

  A. Isolation of group A streptococci

    1. From a sterile site

    2. From a nonsterile site

  B. Clinical signs of severity

    1. Hypotension

    2. At least 2 of the following:

      a. Renal impairment

      b. Coagulopathy

      c. Liver abnormalities

      d. Acute respiratory distress syndrome

      e. Extensive tissue necrosis (eg, necrotizing fasciitis)

      f. Erythematous rash

Staphylococcal TSS[b]

  1. Fever ≥38.9°C

  2. Rash—diffuse, macular erythrodermic

  3. Desquamation—especially on palms and soles, 1-2 wk after onset of illness

  4. Hypotension—SBP <90 mm Hg in adults

  5. Multisystem involvement with ≥3 of the following:

    a. Gastrointestinal tract—vomiting or diarrhea

    b. Muscular—myalgia or elevated creatine kinase

    c. Mucous membranes—vaginal, oropharyngeal, or conjunctival hyperemia

    d. Renal—SUN or creatinine twice the upper limit of reference range

    e. Hepatic—serum bilirubin twice the upper limit of reference range

    f. Hematologic—platelet count <100×10^9/L

    g. CNS—disorientation or alteration in consciousness without focal neurologic signs

  6. Negative results on the following tests:

    a. Blood, throat, or CSF culture (blood culture may be positive for *Staphylococcus aureus*)

    b. Increase in titer for Rocky mountain spotted fever, leptospirosis, or measles

---

Abbreviations: CNS, central nervous system; CSF, cerebrospinal fluid; SBP, systolic blood pressure; SUN, serum urea nitrogen; TSS, toxic shock syndrome.

[a] Definite case: A1 and B1 and B2. Probable case: A2 and B1 and B2.

[b] Probable case: 5 of 6 clinical criteria present. Confirmed case: all 6 clinical criteria present.

Adapted from Silversides JA, Lappin E, Ferguson AJ. Staphylococcal toxic shock syndrome: mechanisms and management. Curr Infect Dis Rep. 2010 Sep;12(5):392-400 and Stevens DL. Streptococcal toxic-shock syndrome: spectrum of disease, pathogenesis, and new concepts in treatment. Emerg Infect Dis. 1995 Jul-Sep;1(3):69-78. Used with permission.

Streptococcal TSS

Although mostly seen with GAS, streptococcal TSS can occur with other groups of β-hemolytic streptococci, such as groups B, C, and G. Risk factors for streptococcal TSS include alcoholism, diabetes mellitus, active varicella infection, and recent surgical procedures. Two factors may contribute to the virulence of GAS. First, a group of proteins (called M proteins; mostly M types 1 and 3) with antiphagocytic properties are expressed on the surface of GAS. Second, streptococcal pyrogenic exotoxins (A, B, and C) can induce cytotoxicity and multiorgan failure. Approximately 80% of GAS strains causing TSS produce pyrogenic exotoxin A. In contrast to staphylococcal TSS that complicates localized infections, streptococcal TSS usually occurs in invasive streptococcal infections, such as necrotizing fasciitis, myonecrosis, or bloodstream infection. Streptococcal infection may also complicate burns, surgical wounds, joint infections, and, rarely, pharyngitis.

Staphylococcal TSS

Two types of staphylococcal TSS exist: menstrual and nonmenstrual. Patients with menstrual TSS usually present within 2 to 3 days of their periods. This typically occurs in patients using tampons (especially with prolonged use of highly absorbent tampons) and is mostly related to TSS toxin-1. Nonmenstrual TSS usually occurs as a complication with wounds (including surgical and postpartum), bone and joint infections, cutaneous infections, and pulmonary infections. Furthermore, it may complicate the use of barrier contraceptive devices.

Treatment of TSS consists of supportive therapy (aggressive fluid resuscitation and vasopressors), surgical débridement of infected sites, removal of tampons (in menstrual TSS), and broad-spectrum antibiotics (which can be de-escalated after the pathogen is confirmed with culture results). Adjunctive clindamycin is recommended to suppress toxin production. Moreover, intravenous immunoglobulin (IVIG) can be used in severe cases that are refractory to standard therapy. Survival benefit of IVIG in streptococcal TSS was seen in an observational study and a small multicenter placebo-controlled trial (4,5). However, the use of IVIG in staphylococcal TSS is less well defined.

In summary, TSS is a toxin-mediated life-threatening illness that requires a high degree of awareness for prompt recognition. The most important management aspect of TSS is to adequately control the source. This often requires surgery for débridement of affected tissues but can be as simple as removing a tampon. All patients with suspected TSS should undergo a thorough physical examination to identify potential sources for drainage or removal. Toxin inhibition or neutralization may be needed in severe cases of TSS.

REFERENCES

1. Schlievert PM. Role of superantigens in human disease. J Infect Dis. 1993 May;167(5): 997–1002.

2. National Notifiable Disease Surveillance System (NNDSS). Streptococcal toxic-shock syndrome (STSS) (*Streptococcus pyogenes*). [updated 2014 May 8; cited 2014 Aug 12]. Atlanta (GA): Centers for Disease Control and Prevention. Available from: http://wwwn.cdc.gov/nndss/script/casedef.aspx?CondYrID=858&DatePub=1/1/2010%2012:00:00%20AM.

3. National Notifiable Disease Surveillance System (NNDSS). Toxic shock syndrome (other than Streptococcal) (TSS). [updated 2014 May 8; cited 2014 Aug 12]. Atlanta (GA): Centers for Disease Control and Prevention. Available from: http://wwwn.cdc.gov/nndss/script/casedef.aspx?CondYrID=869&DatePub=1/1/2011%2012:00:00%20AM.

4. Kaul R, McGeer A, Norrby-Teglund A, Kotb M, Schwartz B, O'Rourke K, et al; The Canadian Streptococcal Study Group. Intravenous immunoglobulin therapy for streptococcal toxic shock syndrome: a comparative observational study. Clin Infect Dis. 1999 Apr;28(4):800–7.

5. Darenberg J, Ihendyane N, Sjolin J, Aufwerber E, Haidl S, Follin P, et al; StreptIg Study Group. Intravenous immunoglobulin G therapy in streptococcal toxic shock syndrome: a European randomized, double-blind, placebo-controlled trial. Clin Infect Dis. 2003 Aug 1;37(3):333–40. Epub 2003 Jul 17.

Diffuse Abdominal Pain in a 45-Year-Old Woman

MAZEN O. AL-QADI, MBBS, JASLEEN R. PANNU, MBBS, AND TENG MOUA, MD

CASE PRESENTATION

A 45-year-old woman with no significant past medical history presented to the emergency department with nausea, vomiting, fever (38.3°C), and diffuse abdominal pain. Physical examination showed respiratory distress with respiratory rate 25 breaths per minute, heart rate 120 beats per minute, blood pressure 90/60 mm Hg, marked epigastric tenderness, and diminished bowel sounds. No scleral icterus was observed. Blood test results are shown in Table 8.1.

Abdominal ultrasonography was negative for biliary stones or signs of cholecystitis. Computed tomography of the abdomen showed moderate peripancreatic edema with no discrete fluid collection. The patient was resuscitated with 4 L of normal saline and began receiving insulin intravenously. A few hours later, she underwent a session of plasmapheresis. She did well and was discharged from the intensive care unit 4 days later without complication.

DISCUSSION

Hypertriglyceridemia-induced pancreatitis is similar in clinical presentation to acute pancreatitis, with abdominal pain, nausea, and vomiting as the most

TABLE 8.1. **Blood Test Results**

Component	Result
Complete blood cell count	Normal
Lipase, U/L	725
Aspartate aminotransferase, U/L	38
Alanine aminotransferase, U/L	32
Alkaline phosphatase, U/L	115
Total bilirubin, mg/dL	0.9
Triglyceride, mg/dL	4,850 (reference range <150)
Glucose, mg/dL	285

common complaints. It is diagnosed from the presence of hypertriglyceridemia (triglycerides >1,000 mg/dL or lipemic serum) and at least 2 of the following features: abdominal pain, elevated serum pancreatic enzymes, or radiographic features of acute pancreatitis in the absence of other causes (eg, gallstones). It is a common cause of acute pancreatitis. The serum amylase level can be falsely low in patients with severe hypertriglyceridemia, so the lipase level should be used instead. Furthermore, a mild elevation of serum triglycerides can be associated with acute pancreatitis from any cause.

The intensivist caring for patients with acute pancreatitis should be aware of the severe complications of acute pancreatitis, including the following (which are not specific for triglycerides-induced pancreatitis):

- Necrosis
- Hemorrhage
- Abdominal compartment syndrome (with aggressively resuscitated patients)
- Gastrointestinal tract bleeding (hemosuccus pancreaticus or gastric varices due to splenic vein thrombosis)
- Pancreatic pseudocyst and abscess
- Acute respiratory distress syndrome
- Severe sepsis

Acute pancreatitis secondary to hypertriglyceridemia should be treated like pancreatitis from other causes, with hydration and analgesia. Postpyloric enteral feeding is associated with favorable outcomes (reduced mortality, fewer infectious complications, reduced need for surgical intervention, and less organ dysfunction) (1). However, hypertriglyceridemia should be controlled before beginning the feeding because of the risk of a further increase in the triglycerides level.

Additionally, hypertriglyceridemia (the triggering factor) should be treated aggressively, with the goal of reducing the serum triglyceride level to less than 500 mg/dL. The following therapeutic approaches have been suggested to achieve this, but no definite guidelines or randomized controlled trials have compared them:

1. In the presence of concomitant hyperglycemia, intravenous insulin with or without intravenous heparin is considered the first choice. Intravenous regular insulin (2) (0.1-0.3 U/kg hourly) is given to maintain the blood glucose level between 150 and 200 mg/dL. It activates lipoprotein lipase and promotes chylomicron degradation, and it is safe in patients with normoglycemia. Intravenous heparin (3) stimulates the release of lipoprotein lipase, but its use is controversial because of its transient effect, with an eventual depletion of lipoprotein lipase stores after an initial increase, and the increased risk of bleeding (eg, hemorrhagic pancreatitis).
2. In the absence of hyperglycemia, plasmapheresis is preferred (4).
3. Lipid-lowering agents (eg, fibrates, ω-3 fatty acids, and statins) are less effective for short-term therapy (they are used mainly for maintenance therapy), they have limited use in patients who cannot tolerate enteral feeding, and they should be initiated as adjuvant therapy as soon as possible.

Patients with hypertriglyceridemia-induced pancreatitis also need to be evaluated for primary dyslipidemia (types I, IV, and V) and secondary hypertriglyceridemia (diabetes mellitus, alcohol, medications, hormonal supplements, pregnancy, and hypothyroidism). Along with exercise, a long-term diet with restrictions for fat and simple sugars is necessary.

REFERENCES

1. Al-Omran M, Albalawi ZH, Tashkandi MF, Al-Ansary LA. Enteral versus parenteral nutrition for acute pancreatitis. Cochrane Database Syst Rev. 2010 Jan 20;(1):CD002837.
2. Mikhail N, Trivedi K, Page C, Wali S, Cope D. Treatment of severe hypertriglyceridemia in nondiabetic patients with insulin. Am J Emerg Med. 2005 May;23(3):415–7.

3. Nasstrom B, Olivecrona G, Olivecrona T, Stegmayr BG. Lipoprotein lipase during continuous heparin infusion: tissue stores become partially depleted. J Lab Clin Med. 2001 Sep;138(3):206–13.

4. Tsuang W, Navaneethan U, Ruiz L, Palascak JB, Gelrud A. Hypertriglyceridemic pancreatitis: presentation and management. Am J Gastroenterol. 2009 Apr;104(4):984–91. Epub 2009 Mar 17.

An Over-the-Counter Intoxication

RONALDO A. SEVILLA BERRIOS, MD, AND KIANOUSH B. KASHANI, MD

CASE PRESENTATION

A 63-year-old woman has a past medical history of chronic obstructive lung disease (she has been receiving long-term oxygen therapy at home), coronary artery disease, and severe rheumatoid arthritis. She presented to her local emergency department with a complaint of generalized weakness and progressive confusion. She had been hospitalized 1 month earlier for an incomplete right acetabular fracture with avascular necrosis of the femur, which was treated conservatively with acetaminophen for pain control. On the initial evaluation she was somnolent but arousable. She was in hypoxemic respiratory failure and required endotracheal intubation and admission to the intensive care unit.

Initial laboratory test results indicated mild anemia; other initial results are shown in Table 9.1.

Results of other studies, including computed tomography of the head, urinalysis, and electrocardiography, were unremarkable. Portable radiography of the chest showed a persistent lung mass in the right lung base. In follow-up computed tomography of the chest, which was done 2 weeks before the latest episode, a well-defined lesion was highly suspicious for malignancy. With gas chromatography–mass spectrometry, the urinary level of 5-oxoproline was 15,805 mmol/mol (reference range ≤62 mmol/mol). Her respiratory status, deemed to be a compensatory mechanism for the underlying metabolic acidosis, improved after 2 days of

TABLE 9.1. Initial Laboratory Test Results

Component	Result
Leukocytes, ×10⁹/L	35
Sodium, mmol/L	141
Potassium, mmol/L	3.8
Chloride, mmol/L	106
Creatinine, mg/dL	1.3
Albumin, g/dL	2.7
Bicarbonate, mmol/L	13
Anion gap	22
Arterial blood gas (after intubation)	
pH	7.21
$Paco_2$, mm Hg	36
Pao_2, mm Hg	139
Base deficit, mEq/L	–13
Lactate, mmol/L	0.6
D-lactate, mmol/L	0.05
Serum osmolality, mOsm/kg	309
β-Hydroxybutyrate, mmol/L	0.1 (reference range <0.4)
Acetaminophen, mg/dL	12
Urine ketones	None

invasive mechanical ventilation; she was extubated successfully, but her overall status did not improve. Owing to her multiple comorbidities, she and her family chose to pursue a palliative-comfort care approach, and she died the next day.

DISCUSSION

Metabolic disarrangements commonly occur in critically ill patients. Since the early 2000s, there has been an increased awareness of the clinically significant complications related to prolonged use and accumulation of acetaminophen metabolites that lead to severe metabolic acidosis with high anion gap (1).

Pyroglutamic acid (5-oxoproline), an infrequent cause of high anion gap metabolic acidosis, was first described in the early 1990s and has gained more recognition since the early 2000s. It can be present with a rare congenital deficit of glutathione synthetase or with an acquired form associated with long-term

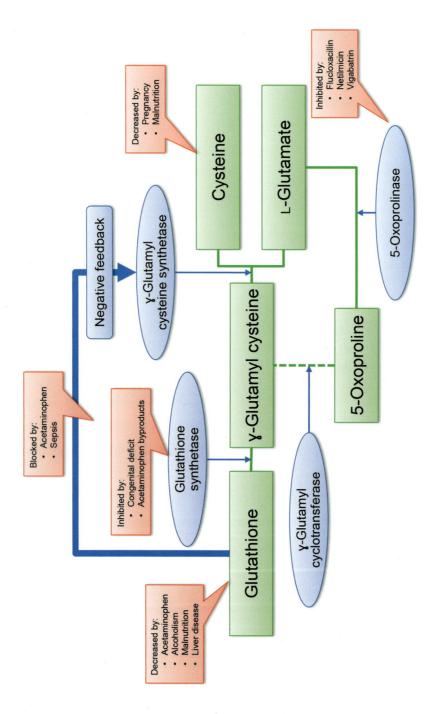

FIGURE 9.1. The γ-Glutamyl Cycle. Acetaminophen, by decreasing glutathione reserves and inhibiting its negative feedback on γ-glutamyl cysteine synthetase, increases γ-glutamyl cysteine and its byproduct, 5-oxoproline. Red boxes list risk factors.

acetaminophen ingestion and malnutrition, severe sepsis, strict vegetarian diet, long-term alcohol consumption, malignancies, pregnancy, and female sex (2). In general, this intoxication is suspected if a patient has metabolic acidosis and a high anion gap that is not explained by the serum lactic acid level, the presence of ketones, alcohol ingestion (abnormal osmolal gap), or renal failure (3). It is understood that 5-oxoproline accumulation occurs because of an absolute or relative deficiency of glutathione synthetase and a subsequent reduction of glutathione levels in the γ-glutamyl cycle (Figure 9.1). This induces accumulation of metabolites and a retrograde inhibition of the pathway, ultimately increasing the levels of 5-oxoproline. With long-term acetaminophen consumption, 1 of the metabolites related to the inhibition of glutathione synthetase function is *N*-acetyl-*p*-benzoquinoneimine (4). Females are at higher risk of this condition developing because they have an increased susceptibility for glutathione synthetase isoenzymes. Other mechanisms for accumulation of 5-oxoproline are summarized in Figure 9.1.

The course is self-limited and the prognosis is generally benign. The main treatment is supportive: Use of the causative agent (eg, acetaminophen or alcohol) is promptly discontinued, or the underlying risk factors (eg, sepsis) are treated (or both steps may be necessary). Severe cases have been successfully treated with *N*-acetylcysteine, particularly in congenital cases in pediatric patients and in adult patients with acetaminophen-induced glutathione synthetase deficiency. *N*-acetylcysteine reestablishes hepatic glutathione storages by providing cysteine that is essential for its synthesis (5).

With the extensive use of acetaminophen, high levels of pyroglutamic acid (5-oxoproline) should be considered when patients with risk factors have an unexplained high anion gap metabolic acidosis. Prompt recognition and withholding acetaminophen are essential in the treatment of this intoxication.

REFERENCES

1. Kortmann W, van Agtmael MA, van Diessen J, Kanen BL, Jakobs C, Nanayakkara PW. 5-Oxoproline as a cause of high anion gap metabolic acidosis: an uncommon cause with common risk factors. Neth J Med. 2008 Sep;66(8):354–7.
2. Fenves AZ, Kirkpatrick HM 3rd, Patel VV, Sweetman L, Emmett M. Increased anion gap metabolic acidosis as a result of 5-oxoproline (pyroglutamic acid): a role for acetaminophen. Clin J Am Soc Nephrol. 2006 May;1(3):441–7. Epub 2006 Apr 19.

3. Liss DB, Paden MS, Schwarz ES, Mullins ME. What is the clinical significance of 5-oxoproline (pyroglutamic acid) in high anion gap metabolic acidosis following paracetamol (acetaminophen) exposure? Clin Toxicol (Phila). 2013 Nov;51(9):817–27. Epub 2013 Oct 11.

4. Esterline RL, Ray SD, Ji S. Reversible and irreversible inhibition of hepatic mitochondrial respiration by acetaminophen and its toxic metabolite, *N*-acetyl-*p*-benzoquinoneimine (NAPQI). Biochem Pharmacol. 1989 Jul 15;38(14):2387–90.

5. Emmett M. Acetaminophen toxicity and 5-oxoproline (pyroglutamic acid): a tale of two cycles, one an ATP-depleting futile cycle and the other a useful cycle. Clin J Am Soc Nephrol. 2014 Jan;9(1):191–200. Epub 2013 Nov 14.

An Over-the-Counter Overdose

MAZEN O. AL-QADI, MBBS,
SARAH B. NELSON, PharmD, RPh,
AND BERNARDO J. SELIM, MD

CASE PRESENTATION

A 19-year-old man with a past medical history significant for depression was admitted after he ingested one hundred 325-mg tablets of enteric-coated aspirin during a suicide attempt. He was taken initially to a local hospital, where an elevated salicylate concentration of 27 mg/dL was measured 4 hours after ingestion. One dose of activated charcoal was given and sodium bicarbonate infusion was initiated. Upon admission to the intensive care unit, physical examination was remarkable for tachycardia, tachypnea, irritability, and diaphoresis. Arterial blood gas results were the following: pH 7.42, $Paco_2$ 37 mm Hg, bicarbonate 24 mmol/L, and Pao_2 64 mm Hg. The salicylate concentration 8 hours later was 42 mg/dL, indicating ongoing absorption. The sodium bicarbonate infusion was continued to maintain a goal urine pH greater than 7.5 for optimal renal clearance of salicylates. Serial salicylate levels were measured every 2 hours until a downward trend was observed, indicating clearance of the drug. The patient improved clinically and never required hemodialysis or ventilatory support.

DISCUSSION

Over-the-counter formulations of salicylates are widely available and exist in the form of acetylsalicylic acid (aspirin), methyl salicylate (wintergreen oil), and bismuth subsalicylate (Pepto-Bismol). In addition, salicylates can be found in combination with other commonly used medications, including antihistamines and narcotics. Approximately 60% of salicylate toxicity is related to acute ingestion. At the cellular level, salicylate toxicity impairs critical metabolic functions through the uncoupling of oxidative phosphorylation and the inhibition of Krebs cycle enzymes and amino acid synthesis, leading to decreased production of adenosine triphosphate. This causes dependence on anaerobic metabolism and consequent lactic acid production and metabolic acidosis. Direct stimulation of the respiratory center causes hyperventilation and respiratory alkalosis (Figure 10.1) (1).

At therapeutic doses, aspirin is readily absorbed in the stomach and small intestine, reaching appreciable blood concentrations within 1 hour after ingestion of a non–enteric-coated formulation and within 4 to 6 hours for an enteric-coated product. When aspirin is taken in large amounts, absorption may be delayed because of drug-induced pylorospasm or bezoar formation. In these instances, peak absorption may not occur for up to 35 hours after ingestion. After absorption, all formulations are hydrolyzed to salicylate (salicylic acid). At physiologic pH, approximately 90% of salicylate is protein bound. It is then metabolized in the liver and excreted in the urine. When aspirin is ingested in supratherapeutic quantities, hepatic conjugation becomes saturated, leaving more unmetabolized salicylate in the blood. The increased concentration of salicylate saturates the available protein-binding sites, ultimately leaving a higher unbound free salicylate concentration available. Free salicylate exists in an ionized form (at physiologic pH) and an un-ionized form (in an acidotic environment). Un-ionized salicylate readily crosses cellular membranes, including the blood-brain barrier, and is responsible for signs of toxicity in salicylate overdose. Renal elimination of salicylate is also impaired, given the saturation of hepatic metabolism preventing the formulation of metabolites that are readily excreted in the urine. This allows for increased reabsorption of un-ionized salicylate in the proximal tubule of the nephron, delaying clearance of the drug from the body.

Acute salicylate toxicity manifests with nonspecific symptoms, including nausea, vomiting, abdominal pain, and tinnitus. Hyperthermia may also occur when energy is dissipated as heat instead of production of adenosine triphosphate. Patients also frequently have tachypnea resulting in respiratory alkalosis, one of the main acid-base disturbances in salicylate toxicity. Severe toxicity may cause other symptoms and clinical signs, including tachycardia, diaphoresis, confusion,

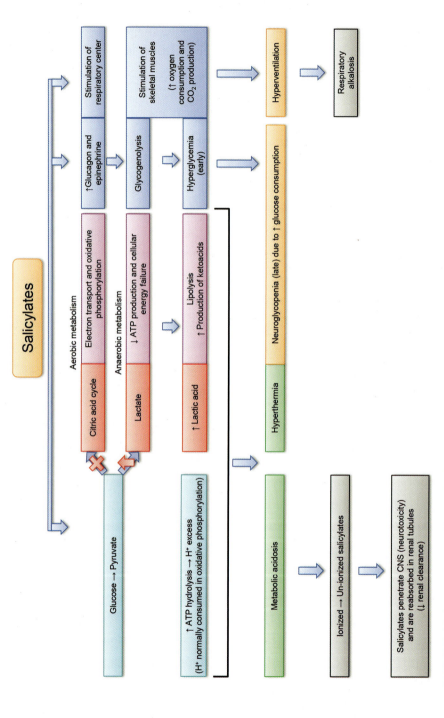

FIGURE 10.1. Metabolic Effects of Salicylates. ATP indicates adenosine triphosphate; CNS, central nervous system; CO_2, carbon dioxide; H^+, hydrogen ion.

seizures, and coma. Noncardiogenic pulmonary edema is a rare but serious complication of salicylate toxicity, although it occurs more often with chronic intoxication (2). Salicylate toxicity also frequently results in hypovolemia due to osmotic diuresis, vomiting, and increased insensible losses (hyperthermia and tachypnea). Acid-base disturbances are a hallmark of salicylate toxicity and follow 3 temporal phases:

1. In the first 12 hours, stimulation of the respiratory center leads to hyperventilation and respiratory alkalosis. This phase is characterized by a compensatory increase in urinary bicarbonate (and potassium) excretion and alkaline urine.
2. From 12 to 24 hours after ingestion, in the presence of continued respiratory alkalosis, renal excretion of hydrogen (due to significant potassium depletion) results in paradoxical aciduria.
3. After 24 hours, the production of hydrogen ions exceeds renal excretion, resulting in metabolic acidosis.

As in any emergency, initial treatment should address airway, breathing, and circulation. Endotracheal intubation in patients with salicylate toxicity may be harmful and should be considered only when the airway is compromised or respiratory failure is clearly present because hypoventilation during the induction period can be fatal (3). Aggressive fluid resuscitation is often required because patients are usually severely hypovolemic. Glucose-containing solutions such as dextrose 5% in water should be used regardless of the serum glucose level to account for decreased cerebral glucose concentrations in salicylate toxicity. This occurs as the rate of cerebral glucose use exceeds the rate of glucose supply (4). Besides supportive care and volume replacement, the main goals of therapy are to minimize absorption, enhance elimination, and minimize penetration of salicylates into the central nervous system. These goals can be achieved by the following:

1. If patients do not have impaired gastric motility, consideration should be given to decontamination of the gastrointestinal tract with single-dose or multiple-dose activated charcoal (25-50 g by mouth every 4 hours for a total of 150 g) to decrease absorption of drug. The benefit of this approach is best when activated charcoal is given within 2 hours after ingestion. When delayed or slow-release product ingestion is suspected, activated charcoal

(>2 hours after ingestion) or whole bowel irrigation should be considered. Although controversial, gastric lavage may also be considered (5).

2. Alkalinization of urine (pH goal >7.5) should be started promptly. Since salicylate is a weak acid, the use of sodium bicarbonate to increase the serum pH above 7.5 promotes the ionization of salicylates, limiting their ability to readily cross cell membranes and decreasing their reabsorption in the proximal tubule of the nephron.

3. Hemodialysis is usually indicated for patients who have evidence of end-organ dysfunction (coma, respiratory failure from pulmonary edema, or renal failure). In addition, hemodialysis is indicated for patients who have high serum salicylate levels (>100 mg/dL in acute intoxication and >40 mg/dL in chronic intoxication).

REFERENCES

1. Tenney SM, Miller RM. The respiratory and circulatory actions of salicylate. Am J Med. 1955 Oct;19(4):498–508.

2. Thisted B, Krantz T, Stroom J, Sorensen MB. Acute salicylate self-poisoning in 177 consecutive patients treated in ICU. Acta Anaesthesiol Scand. 1987 May;31(4):312–6.

3. Stolbach AI, Hoffman RS, Nelson LS. Mechanical ventilation was associated with acidemia in a case series of salicylate-poisoned patients. Acad Emerg Med. 2008 Sep;15(9):866–9.

4. Thurston JH, Pollock PG, Warren SK, Jones EM. Reduced brain glucose with normal plasma glucose in salicylate poisoning. J Clin Invest. 1970 Nov;49(11):2139–45.

5. Juurlink DN, McGuigan MA. Gastrointestinal decontamination for enteric-coated aspirin overdose: what to do depends on who you ask. J Toxicol Clin Toxicol. 2000;38(5):465–70.

A Post–Myocardial Infarction Complication

MAZEN O. AL-QADI, MBBS, AND ERIC L. BLOOMFIELD, MD

CASE PRESENTATION

A 91-year-old man was seen in a local emergency department for retrosternal chest pain followed by syncope. A presumed diagnosis of non–ST-segment elevation myocardial infarction was based on an elevated troponin level without acute changes on electrocardiography (ECG). Treatment was started with aspirin, heparin, and clopidogrel. The patient was then transferred to a tertiary care center, where he underwent a percutaneous coronary intervention for severe lesions in the mid-left anterior descending and mid-right coronary arteries with placement of drug-eluting stents. Two days later, he had acute chest pain followed by circulatory collapse. Cardiopulmonary resuscitation (CPR) was started, and the patient was found to have asystole. During CPR, echocardiography showed pericardial effusion with tamponade. After urgent bedside pericardiocentesis was attempted without success, cardiac surgery was performed. Emergent open pericardectomy through a thoracotomy incision revealed a large blood clot in the pericardium with ongoing active bleeding through a defect in the anterior wall of the left ventricle. After prolonged CPR, and given the poor prognosis, CPR was terminated.

DISCUSSION

Coronary artery disease is a leading cause of death worldwide. Acute myocardial infarction (AMI) can be complicated by arrhythmias, cardiogenic shock, thromboembolism, and inflammatory pericarditis. In addition, several mechanical complications can develop, such as ruptured papillary muscles with acute mitral regurgitation, ventricular septal defect, and free wall rupture. The introduction of percutaneous coronary intervention after AMI has reduced the incidence and shifted the timing of these complications.

Ventricular free wall rupture (VFWR) is a rare catastrophic complication that develops in 0.5% of patients after AMI and carries a mortality rate of 20% (1). However, VFWR is found in 14% to 26% of patients who die after AMI. Other causes of VFWR include device implantation, myocardial abscess, cardiac tumors, aortic dissection, and cardiac surgery. Moreover, myocardial rupture has been reported to occur with takotsubo cardiomyopathy (2). Although free wall rupture usually involves the left ventricle, right ventricular rupture has been reported. Most VFWR cases (90%) occur in the first 2 weeks after AMI, with about 50% occurring within the first 5 days after AMI. The left anterior descending and circumflex coronary arteries are the culprit vessels in 80% of cases.

The following risk factors are associated with increased risk of VFWR: female sex, older age (>60 years), long-standing hypertension, single-vessel disease, first lateral or anterior wall AMI, persistent ST-segment elevation on ECG, presence of Q wave on the initial ECG, and transmural infarction. Despite earlier reports of a possible association between corticosteroid therapy and VFWR, a meta-analysis of 11 controlled trials showed no association with corticosteroid therapy (3). Furthermore, delayed use of a fibrinolytic agent was not associated with an increased risk of VFWR. However, late fibrinolysis may accelerate rupture to within 24 hours of treatment (4). In addition, early administration of β-blockers and angiotensin-converting enzyme inhibitors (when appropriate) can be protective against myocardial rupture.

Four distinct types of VFWR have been described:

- Type I (occurs <24 hours post–myocardial infarction [MI]) is a small, abrupt, full-thickness tear without thinning. It occurs mostly in patients receiving thrombolytic therapy.

- Type II (occurs 1-3 days post-MI) is an erosion of the infarcted segment in multiple directions with bloody infiltrate.
- Type III (occurs >3 days post-MI) is a rupture of the ventricular wall due to thinning of the border zone of the infarction and normal myocardium. This type results from dynamic left ventricular outflow tract obstruction and increased ventricular wall stress with aneurysm formation. The opening of a type III rupture is usually protected by a thrombus or the pericardium.
- Type IV (no specific time frame has been described) is an incomplete rupture (ie, without extension through all layers of the myocardium).

Clinically, patients may feel acute chest pain after coughing or straining. Type I VFWR produces a sudden cardiovascular collapse followed by electromechanical dissociation due to hemopericardium and tamponade. Bleeding may stop if a blood clot forms and seals the pericardial leak. One-third of patients may have slow repetitive bleeding and survive until they undergo emergent surgical repair. Patients with type II or III VFWR usually present with refractory cardiogenic shock. Overall, VFWR is associated with a mortality rate of 20%. If VFWR is suspected, transthoracic echocardiography should be used to confirm the diagnosis as soon as possible. Transthoracic echocardiography is the most sensitive diagnostic modality that is readily available for a timely diagnosis. It may show pericardial effusion or signs of tamponade (right-sided cardiac collapse, dilatation of the inferior vena cava, and marked respiratory variation in mitral and tricuspid valve inflow) and possibly a cardiac defect at the rupture site. In the presence of a pulmonary artery catheter, signs of tamponade (equalization of right atrial, right ventricular diastolic, and pulmonary capillary wedge pressures) can be evident.

Treatment should start with fluid resuscitation to increase cardiac filling and inotropes to improve cardiac output. Vasopressors can also be used to achieve hemodynamic stability. Immediate pericardiocentesis is used to stabilize the patient hemodynamically until surgical intervention is performed. Although controversial, an intra-aortic balloon pump can be used in patients with free wall rupture as a bridge to surgery (5). Emergent surgical intervention, the only definitive therapy, consists of repair of the defect with or without excising the infarcted myocardium (ie, infarctectomy).

VFWR is a rare and potentially fatal complication after MI. Manifestations vary, depending on whether the VFWR occurs in the first day after MI, in the second or third day after MI, or later. Emergent surgery is the only definitive therapy.

REFERENCES

1. French JK, Hellkamp AS, Armstrong PW, Cohen E, Kleiman NS, O'Connor CM, et al. Mechanical complications after percutaneous coronary intervention in ST-elevation myocardial infarction (from APEX-AMI). Am J Cardiol. 2010 Jan 1;105(1):59–63.

2. Kumar S, Kaushik S, Nautiyal A, Choudhary SK, Kayastha BL, Mostow N, et al. Cardiac rupture in takotsubo cardiomyopathy: a systematic review. Clin Cardiol. 2011 Nov;34(11):672–6. Epub 2011 Sep 14.

3. Giugliano GR, Giugliano RP, Gibson CM, Kuntz RE. Meta-analysis of corticosteroid treatment in acute myocardial infarction. Am J Cardiol. 2003 May 1;91(9):1055–9.

4. Becker RC, Charlesworth A, Wilcox RG, Hampton J, Skene A, Gore JM, et al. Cardiac rupture associated with thrombolytic therapy: impact of time to treatment in the Late Assessment of Thrombolytic Efficacy (LATE) study. J Am Coll Cardiol. 1995 Apr;25(5):1063–8.

5. Pifarre R, Sullivan HJ, Grieco J, Montoya A, Bakhos M, Scanlon PJ, et al. Management of left ventricular rupture complicating myocardial infarction. J Thorac Cardiovasc Surg. 1983 Sep;86(3):441–3.

Massive Hemoptysis

MAZEN O. AL-QADI, MBBS, AND MARK E. WYLAM, MD

CASE PRESENTATION

A 50-year-old woman with metastatic adenoid cystic carcinoma involving the trachea was transferred to the intensive care unit after cardiopulmonary arrest due to acute hemoptysis. Upon admission to the ward, she had another episode of massive hemoptysis (>500 mL) and became unresponsive. Cardiopulmonary resuscitation (CPR) was initiated because she was pulseless. When endotracheal intubation was performed, she had a substantial amount of blood in the upper airway. After 2 minutes of CPR, spontaneous circulation returned.

The patient's past medical history was significant for radiotherapy to the tracheal tumor 5 years before this admission. Two prior episodes of hemoptysis had resulted in emergent bronchoscopy and placement of tracheal stents. During the first episode, a covered self-expandable metallic stent was placed over the tumor bed. During the second episode, the stent was partially obstructed with tumor at its proximal and distal ends by a combination of malignancy and granulation tissue. Thus, silastic stents were deployed within both the distal end and the proximal end of the preexisting stent with good endoscopic results. Presently, with an endotracheal tube in place, airway bleeding appeared controlled. This created the suspicion that the proximal aspect of the wire mesh stent had eroded into the innominate artery, causing the massive hemoptysis.

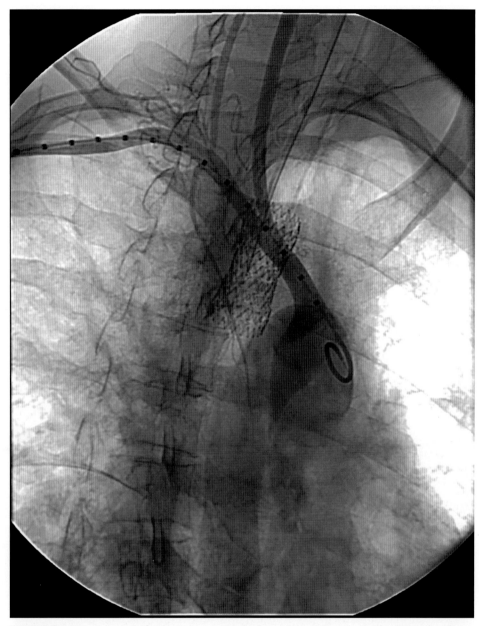

FIGURE 12.1. Stent Graft Placement in Right Innominate Artery. Marker pigtail catheter was advanced and placed in the ascending thoracic aorta. Endotracheal tube and balloon within wire mesh tracheal stent are visible. Wire mesh stent is shown overlying the innominate artery with no evidence of pseudoaneurysm or active bleeding. Later, an 8×38-mm iCAST covered stent (Atrium Medical Corp) was placed to cover the entire innominate artery from its origin to its bifurcation.

Immediately, an interventional radiology team placed an 8.0-mm stent graft into the right innominate artery overlying the wire mesh stent from its origin to its bifurcation (Figure 12.1). The patient had no further bleeding and was successfully extubated to receive palliative care.

DISCUSSION

Massive hemoptysis is a life-threatening condition that accounts for 5% to 10% of all cases of hemoptysis. Although rapid bleeding of 100 to 200 mL of blood (equivalent to the anatomical dead space) can compromise upper airways and impair gas exchange, expectoration of more than 600 mL of blood in 24 hours is the commonly used definition of *massive hemoptysis*. This definition, however, does not account for important clinical variables such as the patient's ability to maintain the airway patency, the rate of bleeding, and the presence of cardiopulmonary comorbidities (1).

The most common causes of massive hemoptysis are bronchiectasis, tuberculosis (most common in developing countries), mycetoma, transbronchial biopsy, necrotizing pneumonia, bronchogenic carcinoma, and fibrosing mediastinitis (Box 12.1). Bleeding typically originates from 1 of the following sources: 1) branches of the systemic pressure bronchial vessels (90% of massive hemoptysis cases); 2) systemic pressure nonbronchial vessels (5% of cases) (eg, tracheoinnominate fistula from tracheostomy, or aortotracheal aneurysm); or 3) pulmonary pressure circulation (5% of cases) (eg, pulmonary vasculitis, pulmonary infarction, pulmonary artery aneurysm, or arteriovenous malformations).

The primary cause of death in massive hemoptysis is asphyxia. Therefore, interventions should focus on securing the airway, containing and controlling the bleeding by isolation of the bleeding side, and, occasionally, providing hemodynamic stabilization.

BOX 12.1.
ETIOLOGY OF MASSIVE HEMOPTYSIS

Central (airways): endobronchial tumors, trauma, or tracheoarterial fistula

Distal (airways or parenchyma): bronchiectasis, tuberculosis, mycetoma, or necrotizing pneumonia

Vascular: pulmonary artery rupture or aneurysm, pulmonary infarct, pulmonary hypertension, or pulmonary arteriovenous malformation

Coagulopathy: rare cause in the absence of procedures or interventions

Posttracheostomy

  Early (within hours): perioperative coagulopathy or inadequate surgical homeostasis

  Late (days to weeks): most (75%) are due to tracheoinnominate fistula and are often heralded by a self-limited sentinel bleed several hours before massive bleeding

---

Patients with hemodynamic instability or respiratory compromise need to be intubated as soon as possible. A large-caliber endotracheal tube (internal diameter ≥8 mm) should be used to facilitate adequate suctioning and further interventions. It may be advanced in the main bronchus of the unaffected lung to isolate the bleeding side.

When the bleeding side is known, the patient should be positioned on the same side (with the affected lung in a gravity-dependent position) to limit the spread of blood to the contralateral unaffected lung.

Bronchoscopy is the most effective tool for clearing blood clots (2). It may be used to isolate the unaffected lung and to intervene to control bleeding in 1 of 2 ways: 1) Selectively intubate the unaffected lung. This method is not preferred for bleeding in the left lung, since intubating the right lung will result in occlusion of the right upper lobe bronchus and will further compromise gas exchange. 2) Contain the bleeding with a bronchial block with either a Fogarty balloon catheter or a pulmonary artery balloon catheter. A Fogarty balloon catheter can be used for main, lobar, and segmental bronchi and can stay in place for up to 1 week (deflated for a few minutes 3 times daily to preserve mucosal viability). The risk of pneumonia increases when the catheter is left in place for 5 days. When the placement of an endobronchial block during active bleeding is difficult because of poor visualization of the airway, placement under fluoroscopy is preferred. A pulmonary artery balloon catheter can be used to occlude more distal segments and to optimize gas exchange.

Local administration of agents to control bleeding, such as cold saline irrigation and vasoconstrictive agents, can also be attempted. The vasoconstrictors epinephrine and vasopressin are useful in mild to moderate bleeding but may cause systemic adverse effects, such as hypertension and arrhythmia, so their use is discouraged. The use of tranexamic acid, an antifibrinolytic, has been described in case reports; this agent may be used to achieve hemostasis in cases refractory to cold saline and epinephrine. Fibrinogen-thrombin with or without factor XIII, recombinant activated factor VII (rFVIIa), and aprotinin form a stable fibrin clot and can stop the bleeding promptly but are associated with rebleeding; therefore, they are used as a temporary measure before definitive therapy (3,4). rFVIIa has also been used endobronchially.

Advanced interventions (eg, stents, cryoprobe) are usually performed by an interventional pulmonologist for central airway bleeding (usually with rigid bronchoscopy) and are beyond the scope of this review.

Definitive therapy may be either endovascular or surgical intervention. Endovascular therapy (ie, bronchial artery embolization) can be performed after the patient's condition is stabilized. This procedure carries a small risk of neurologic damage (5% of the population has a spinal artery that originates from a bronchial artery). However, this risk has been minimized by using the superselective catheters to embolize the bronchial artery more distally (5). Surgical interventions are indicated when endovascular intervention fails to control the patient's bleeding. These patients almost always have massive hemoptysis due to mycetoma.

REFERENCES

1. Ibrahim WH. Massive haemoptysis: the definition should be revised. Eur Respir J. 2008 Oct;32(4):1131–2.

2. Dweik RA, Stoller JK. Role of bronchoscopy in massive hemoptysis. Clin Chest Med. 1999 Mar;20(1):89–105.

3. de Gracia J, de la Rosa D, Catalan E, Alvarez A, Bravo C, Morell F. Use of endoscopic fibrinogen-thrombin in the treatment of severe hemoptysis. Respir Med. 2003 Jul;97(7):790–5.

4. Heslet L, Nielsen JD, Levi M, Sengelov H, Johansson PI. Successful pulmonary administration of activated recombinant factor VII in diffuse alveolar hemorrhage. Crit Care. 2006;10(6):R177.

5. Mal H, Rullon I, Mellot F, Brugiere O, Sleiman C, Menu Y, et al. Immediate and long-term results of bronchial artery embolization for life-threatening hemoptysis. Chest. 1999 Apr;115(4):996–1001.

Hypotension Following a Broken Hip

JOSEPH H. SKALSKI, MD, AND DARYL J. KOR, MD

CASE PRESENTATION

A 55-year-old man with an unremarkable past medical history sustained a left acetabular fracture after an injury at a construction site. He was admitted to the hospital and underwent uncomplicated open reduction and internal fixation of the hip fracture. During a rehabilitation session 1 day after the surgical procedure, he had an abrupt onset of cyanosis, shortness of breath, and diaphoresis. The emergency response team was activated, but the patient's condition rapidly deteriorated, and he became pulseless and unresponsive. Chest compressions were provided, Advanced Cardiovascular Life Support resuscitation was initiated, and the patient was intubated uneventfully. After 12 minutes of cardiopulmonary resuscitation, including 2 defibrillations, spontaneous circulation returned, and he was transferred to the intensive care unit for further management.

Upon arrival in the intensive care unit, the patient had a palpable pulse but remained hypotensive, tachycardic, and unresponsive. Intravenous vasoactive medications were initiated to maintain adequate blood pressure. Intravenous heparin therapy was started out of concern for acute pulmonary embolism. After the patient's condition was stable, computed tomographic angiography of the chest was performed and confirmed the finding of massive pulmonary embolism (Figure 13.1). Transthoracic echocardiography subsequently showed severe right ventricular dilatation, decreased right ventricular systolic function, and

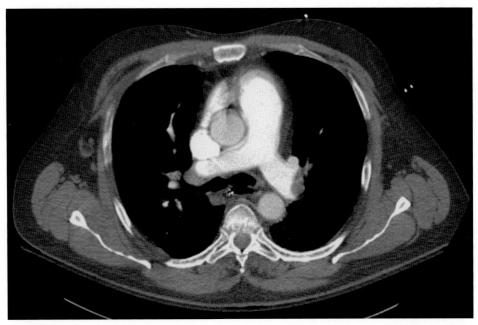

FIGURE 13.1. Pulmonary Embolism. Computed tomographic chest angiogram shows bilateral central pulmonary emboli involving the right and distal left main pulmonary arteries.

an underfilled left ventricular cavity with preserved systolic function. Systemic thrombolytic therapy was not administered because of the patient's recent surgery. After a cardiovascular surgery consultation, the patient was not thought to be a good candidate for surgical thromboembolectomy because of the peripheral distribution of the emboli.

Over the subsequent days, his hemodynamic status improved, and the vasoactive infusions were stopped. His respiratory status also improved, so that his ventilator was used to provide only minimal support. Despite his cardiopulmonary improvement, the patient remained comatose. Magnetic resonance imaging of the head showed evidence of severe anoxic brain injury, which was likely sustained during his cardiac arrest. After discussion with the patient's family, a neurologist, and the palliative medicine team, the patient's medical decision-maker elected for comfort-directed care. Ventilator support was withdrawn, and the patient died peacefully in the presence of his family.

DISCUSSION

Anticoagulant medications are the mainstay of therapy for acute pulmonary embolism (1). Parenteral anticoagulants, such as heparin, should be initiated immediately in patients presenting with acute pulmonary embolism unless there is a specific contraindication. In patients with a high clinical suspicion for pulmonary embolism and no contraindications to pharmacologic anticoagulation, therapy should be initiated without delay—even before confirmatory diagnostic testing (1).

As this patient's story illustrates, poor outcomes can occur in acute pulmonary embolism even with appropriate anticoagulant therapy. Systemic thrombolytic therapy has been studied as a way to improve outcomes in acute pulmonary embolism. Thrombolytic therapies such as recombinant tissue plasminogen activator or streptokinase activate plasmin, thereby promoting fibrin degradation (1). These therapies are typically administered as a single short infusion at the time of diagnosis of pulmonary embolism. Importantly, thrombolytic therapy is not a substitute for appropriate anticoagulation (1). Thrombolytic therapy results in accelerated lysis of thrombus and thus has theoretical benefit in the treatment of acute pulmonary embolus. However, the risk of major bleeding is increased with thrombolytic administration compared to anticoagulation alone, and multiple studies have shown no mortality benefit with thrombolytic therapy in unselected patients with acute pulmonary embolism (1,2).

Massive pulmonary embolism is defined as a pulmonary embolus resulting in shock or hypotension. Patients with massive pulmonary embolus have a high risk of death, and thus they may be expected to have the most to gain from systemic thrombolysis. The role of thrombolytic therapy in massive pulmonary embolism has not been examined in a large randomized trial. However, a retrospective national database review of 72,230 patients with unstable pulmonary embolus identified a 47% mortality rate for patients receiving no thrombolytic therapy compared to a 15% mortality rate for patients who received thrombolytics (3). Furthermore, the 2012 (9th edition) American College of Chest Physicians (ACCP) guidelines recommend the administration of systemic thrombolytic therapy in patients with massive pulmonary embolism, provided there are no contraindications (1).

A challenging scenario often encountered by clinicians is a patient without shock but with right ventricular dysfunction on echocardiography, an elevated troponin level, or a large clot burden on imaging. The Moderate Pulmonary Embolism Treated With Thrombolysis (MOPETT) trial examined reduced-dose thrombolytic therapy for patients with right ventricular dysfunction or more than 70% involvement of the pulmonary arteries with thrombus on imaging (4). There was no statistically significant reduction in clinical end points, such as mortality or recurrent pulmonary embolism, but patients randomly assigned to receive thrombolytics did have a sustained reduction in pulmonary artery pressures on echocardiography (4). Further research is needed to determine which patients with submassive pulmonary embolism may benefit from systemic thrombolytic therapy. The current (9th edition) ACCP guidelines do not explicitly recommend systemic thrombolytics for patients with submassive pulmonary embolism with right ventricular dysfunction or elevated troponin.

The patient in this case presented with massive pulmonary embolism and thus was a candidate for thrombolytic administration. However, his recent surgical procedure (<24 hours earlier) was thought to be a contraindication to thrombolytic therapy, so this treatment was not provided.

Anticoagulant medications such as heparin are the mainstay of therapy for pulmonary embolism and should be initiated as early as possible in patients who have no contraindications and a high clinical suspicion for pulmonary embolism. Systemic thrombolytic therapy should be administered to patients with shock due to pulmonary embolism (ie, massive pulmonary embolism) if there are no contraindications. The role of systemic thrombolytic therapy in other disorders, such as submassive pulmonary embolism, is poorly defined and requires further research.

REFERENCES

1. Kearon C, Akl EA, Comerota AJ, Prandoni P, Bounameaux H, Goldhaber SZ, et al; American College of Chest Physicians. Antithrombotic therapy for VTE disease: antithrombotic therapy and prevention of thrombosis, 9th ed: American College of Chest Physicians Evidence-Based Clinical Practice guidelines. Chest. 2012 Feb;141(2 Suppl):e419S-94S. Erratum in: Chest. 2012 Dec;142(6):1698–704.

2. Wan S, Quinlan DJ, Agnelli G, Eikelboom JW. Thrombolysis compared with heparin for the initial treatment of pulmonary embolism: a meta-analysis of the randomized controlled trials. Circulation. 2004 Aug 10;110(6):744–9. Epub 2004 Jul 19.

3. Stein PD, Matta F. Thrombolytic therapy in unstable patients with acute pulmonary embolism: saves lives but underused. Am J Med. 2012 May;125(5):465–70. Epub 2012 Feb 10. Erratum in: Am J Med. 2012 Jul;125(7):e13.

4. Sharifi M, Bay C, Skrocki L, Rahimi F, Mehdipour M; "MOPETT" Investigators. Moderate pulmonary embolism treated with thrombolysis (from the "MOPETT" trial). Am J Cardiol. 2013 Jan 15;111(2):273–7. Epub 2012 Oct 24.

Extubation Failure

MUHAMMAD A. RISHI, MBBS, AND NATHAN J. SMISCHNEY, MD

CASE PRESENTATION

A 74-year-old woman was admitted with a past medical history significant for type 2 diabetes mellitus, peptic ulcer disease, hypertension, coronary artery disease with a positive exercise stress test 2 weeks before admission (with inferior myocardial ischemia noted at a heart rate of 116 beats per minute but a preserved ejection fraction of 60%), and an L1 intradural schwannoma. On the day of admission, she underwent L1 laminectomy and resection of the tumor. She was intubated with a 7-mm cuffed endotracheal tube. Her intraoperative course was unremarkable. She received 2 L of crystalloid and lost an estimated 50 mL of blood.

She was extubated and hemodynamically stable when she was transferred to the postanesthesia care unit (PACU). However, in the PACU, she was somnolent and was noted to have frequent obstructive apneic events and snoring. She became progressively hypoxic and cyanotic. She was treated with noninvasive ventilation (NIV). She initially responded to NIV but subsequently became more hypoxic. Arterial blood gas measurements were pH 7.31, Pco_2 57 mm Hg, and Po_2 57 mm Hg. On chest radiography, diffuse infiltrates throughout both lungs were greatest in the perihilar regions and consistent with pulmonary edema (Figure 14.1). An electrocardiogram did not show any change from a previous one, and initial and subsequent troponin levels were within the reference range. Emergent

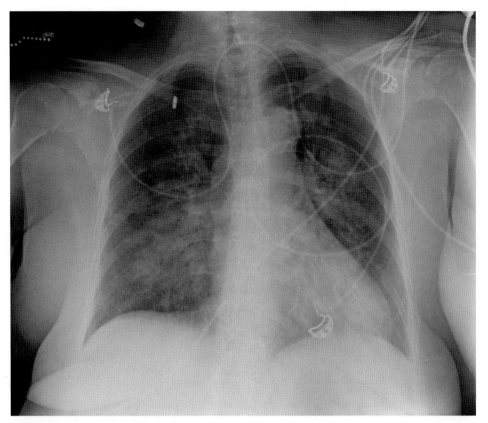

FIGURE 14.1. Pulmonary Edema. This chest radiograph is from a patient who had negative pressure pulmonary edema after extubation.

echocardiography showed a normal ejection fraction and hyperdynamic ventricles. Since the patient did not improve with NIV, she was promptly reintubated. She was extubated 6 hours later without difficulty.

DISCUSSION

Negative pressure pulmonary edema (NPPE) is an uncommon, potentially life-threatening complication of general anesthesia, occurring in about 0.1% of cases (1). It is a process marked by transudation of fluid into the pulmonary interstitium as a result of markedly negative intrathoracic pressure (1). Although various causes have been suggested, postextubation stridor, unrecognized sleep apnea, and strangulation or hanging are the most common.

NPPE characteristically develops after upper airway obstruction. The entity occurs in patients of all ages but typically occurs in middle-aged men. Factors that may predispose to NPPE are short neck, difficult intubation, endotracheal tube obstruction, history of obstructive sleep apnea, obesity, acromegaly, and upper airway surgery. Two forms of NPPE have been described: Type 1 characteristically develops when there is immediate upper airway obstruction (eg, postextubation laryngospasm), and type 2 develops after release of chronic airway obstruction (eg, after resection of an upper airway tumor) (2).

The pathophysiology of NPPE is marked by development of negative intrathoracic pressure against a closed glottis (modified Müller maneuver) causing very negative pleural pressures. The result is movement of blood to the pulmonary vascular bed, leading to an increase in pulmonary hydrostatic pressure and a subsequent fluid leak from the pulmonary microcirculation. Hypoxia-induced pulmonary vasoconstriction and reduced pulmonary interstitial pressure cause further worsening of the pulmonary edema. A secondary mechanism may be release of catecholamines as a result of stress. This adrenergic surge causes an increased left ventricular afterload and a diminishing left-sided ejection fraction; the result is an increase in left ventricular end-systolic and end-diastolic volumes and pulmonary edema (3).

Often NPPE develops within minutes and resolves within 24 to 36 hours. Use of diuretics is controversial. Infrequently, only supplemental oxygen suffices. Mechanical ventilation is the mainstay of treatment; however, continuous positive airway pressure or bilevel positive airway pressure can be used under certain situations (4). Pulmonary hemorrhage is a rare complication of NPPE (2).

NPPE is an important cause of morbidity, unexpected intensive care admission, and, occasionally, mortality among postoperative patients. It is a well described and probably underrecognized clinical syndrome. Early recognition of the condition is the key, allowing for prompt application of positive airway pressure and rapid resolution of the condition.

REFERENCES

1. Tami TA, Chu F, Wildes TO, Kaplan M. Pulmonary edema and acute upper airway obstruction. Laryngoscope. 1986 May;96(5):506–9.
2. Schwartz DR, Maroo A, Malhotra A, Kesselman H. Negative pressure pulmonary hemorrhage. Chest. 1999 Apr;115(4):1194–7.

3. Koh MS, Hsu AA, Eng P. Negative pressure pulmonary oedema in the medical intensive care unit. Intensive Care Med. 2003 Sep;29(9):1601–4. Epub 2003 Jul 17.

4. Furuichi M, Takeda S, Akada S, Onodera H, Yoshida Y, Nakazato K, et al. Noninvasive positive pressure ventilation in patients with perioperative negative pressure pulmonary edema. J Anesth. 2010 Jun;24(3):464–8. Epub 2010 Mar 11.

Hypotension and Right-Sided Heart Failure After Left Pneumonectomy

MISTY A. RADOSEVICH, MD,
W. BRIAN BEAM, MD,
AND ONUR DEMIRCI, MD

CASE PRESENTATION

A 65-year-old man with a history of coronary artery disease and malignant mesothelioma, for which he has received chemotherapy, underwent left pneumonectomy for operative management of the malignancy. After an uneventful induction, he was intubated with a left-sided double-lumen endotracheal tube. A left pneumonectomy was performed through a left posterolateral thoracotomy; a large pericardiectomy was electively not repaired. A chest tube was placed and set to water seal. The patient was extubated in the operating room and was taken to the postanesthesia care unit (PACU).

Shortly after arrival in the PACU, the patient had significant hypotension (systolic blood pressure about 40 mm Hg) when his position was changed. He required multiple boluses of phenylephrine, ephedrine, and epinephrine and ultimately a phenylephrine infusion. An electrocardiogram (ECG) showed new non-specific ST-segment and T-wave abnormalities in the anterolateral leads and a new incomplete right bundle branch block. Transthoracic echocardiography showed a hyperdynamic D-shaped left ventricle with an ejection fraction of 70%. No regional wall motion abnormalities were noted, but the patient had moderate-to-severe right ventricular dilatation and severe tricuspid regurgitation with a right ventricular systolic pressure of 54 mm Hg (systolic blood pressure 122 mm Hg). A chest radiograph showed only the expected postpneumonectomy changes. The troponin T level was moderately elevated, and the hemoglobin concentration was mildly decreased from preoperative values.

Throughout, the patient reported no chest pain, chest pressure, or shortness of breath, but he had an episode of unresponsiveness during a hypotensive period after transfer to the intensive care unit (ICU). Norepinephrine, vasopressin, and milrinone were added for hemodynamic support. Phenylephrine was discontinued. The elevated troponin levels trended downward. The following day, an ECG showed right-axis deviation and an $S_1Q_3T_3$ pattern. A computed tomographic (CT) angiogram with a pulmonary embolus protocol was negative for emboli. However, the heart had shifted significantly to the left, and the right pulmonary artery (PA) appeared to be markedly narrowed approximately 2.4 cm above the pulmonary valve (Figure 15.1). The patient was taken back to the operating room, where his heart was found to have herniated through the unrepaired pericardial defect. As a result of the heart protruding through this defect, an edge of pericardium was compressing the main PA. After the heart was repositioned within the pericardial sac, intraoperative transesophageal echocardiography showed resolution of the PA obstruction and improved right-sided heart dynamics. The pericardial defect was closed with bovine pericardial mesh.

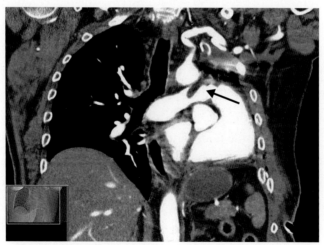

FIGURE 15.1. Compression of Pulmonary Artery. Coronal computed tomographic image shows a leftward shift of the heart and compression of the pulmonary artery by an edge of pericardium (arrow).

The patient was extubated in the immediate postoperative period. Less than 12 hours later, all vasopressor support was discontinued. Two days after reoperation, the patient was transferred from the ICU; he was discharged home on hospital day 8.

DISCUSSION

Cardiac herniation is a rare but serious complication that may develop after pneumonectomy. It occurs when the heart is displaced through a pericardial defect into the newly empty hemithorax. Between 1951 and 2005, approximately 50 cases of postpneumonectomy cardiac herniation were reported (1). However, a higher incidence (3%) has been described for extrapleural pneumonectomy in patients who have had chemotherapy for malignant mesothelioma (2). The majority of cases occur in the immediate postoperative period, and nearly all occur within the first 24 hours. Signs and symptoms are nonspecific, and cardiac herniation requires a high degree of awareness because the mortality is 100% if the herniation is unrecognized and untreated; even when it is recognized and treated rapidly, 50% mortality has been reported (1).

Cardiac herniation is challenging to diagnose given its nonspecific presentation. In addition, signs and symptoms differ depending on the side of herniation. The physiologic perturbations seen with right-sided herniations result from rotation of the heart and venae cavae leading to impaired venous return to the right side of the heart and superior vena cava syndrome (3). The presentation of left-sided herniations is typically secondary to strangulation of the ventricles by the pericardium, leading to impaired perfusion of the ventricular wall and related sequelae (eg, arrhythmias, outflow tract obstruction, and myocardial ischemia) (1).

Factors that predispose to cardiac herniation include negative pressure in the intrathoracic space (eg, suction applied to the empty hemithorax), rolling the patient so the operative side is dependent, aggressive positive pressure ventilation, and violent coughing bouts (1,3).

Unlike right-sided herniations, in which the heart is seen in the right hemithorax, left-sided herniations are not obvious on chest radiography. The appearance of left-sided cardiac herniations on chest radiography are subtle and have been described as a left shift of the cardiac shadow, resulting in better visualization of the spine with a round, poorly defined opacity representing the herniated portion of the heart (3).

Echocardiography, described as a useful tool in diagnosis of cardiac herniation, shows a mass effect on the heart by the pericardial edges (1). However, this was not evident in the echocardiographic images for the patient in the present case.

Although CT imaging was very helpful in the present case, the utility of CT in the diagnosis of this entity is not well described. However, it has been shown to be a useful tool to diagnose pericardial rupture and subsequent cardiac herniation after blunt chest trauma (4).

Management centers on emergent operative repair, but conservative measures have been suggested to improve stability until the patient is returned to the operating room. These measures include positioning the patient with the nonoperative side down, avoiding aggressive positive pressure ventilation, and injecting air into the empty hemithorax (5).

Cardiac herniation is a diagnostic challenge. Because early recognition and intervention are critical to the survival of these patients, a high degree of awareness of this condition is necessary when hypotensive patients have undergone pneumonectomy involving pericardiectomy.

REFERENCES

1. Chambers N, Walton S, Pearce A. Cardiac herniation following pneumonectomy: an old complication revisited. Anaesth Intensive Care. 2005 Jun;33(3):403–9.

2. Opitz I, Kestenholz P, Lardinois D, Muller M, Rousson V, Schneiter D, et al. Incidence and management of complications after neoadjuvant chemotherapy followed by extrapleural pneumonectomy for malignant pleural mesothelioma. Eur J Cardiothorac Surg. 2006 Apr;29(4): 579–84. Epub 2006 Feb 21.

3. Yacoub MH, Williams WG, Ahmad A. Strangulation of the heart following intrapericardial pneumonectomy. Thorax. 1968 May;23(3):261–5.

4. Schir F, Thony F, Chavanon O, Perez-Moreira I, Blin D, Coulomb M. Blunt traumatic rupture of the pericardium with cardiac herniation: two cases diagnosed using computed tomography. Eur Radiol. 2001;11(6):995–9.

5. Cassorla L, Katz JA. Management of cardiac herniation after intrapericardial pneumonectomy. Anesthesiology. 1984 Apr;60(4):362–4.

More Than Meets the Eye

SUMEDH S. HOSKOTE, MBBS, SHIVANI S. SHINDE, MBBS, AND NATHAN J. SMISCHNEY, MD

CASE PRESENTATION

An 80-year-old man with aortic stenosis that was repaired with a bioprosthetic valve is morbidly obese and has severe obesity-hypoventilation syndrome that is treated with nocturnal mechanical ventilation through a tracheostomy. He presented to the emergency department at a community hospital with worsening dyspnea for a few days and was found to have a severely elevated leukocyte count of 247×10^9/L. He was transferred to a tertiary care center for further management for a presumptive diagnosis of leukemia with blast crisis.

On arrival, the patient was being mechanically ventilated through a tracheostomy and had an intraosseous line to administer norepinephrine for blood pressure support. Notable vital signs were temperature 36.8°C, heart rate 124 beats per minute, blood pressure 97/42 mm Hg (mean arterial pressure 55 mm Hg), respiratory rate 20 breaths per minute, and oxygen saturation 98% with 100% oxygen. On physical examination, the patient was a morbidly obese man who weighed 143 kg and was deeply comatose (Glasgow Coma Score, 3 of 15), with a thready pulse and coarse bilateral breath sounds. Cardiac monitoring showed sinus tachycardia. Laboratory test results were urgently obtained (Table 16.1). Arterial blood gas results were pH 6.85, $Paco_2$ 74 mm Hg, Pao_2 51 mm Hg, and

TABLE 16.1. **Laboratory Test Results**

Component	Result	Reference
Sodium, mmol/L	138	135–145
Chloride, mmol/L	99	100–108
Potassium, mmol/L	5.0	3.6–5.2
Bicarbonate, mmol/L	16	22–29
Serum urea nitrogen, mg/dL	28	6–21
Creatinine, mg/dL	3.3	0.7–1.2
Inorganic phosphorous, mg/dL	7.9	2.5–4.5
Calcium, mg/dL	9.2	8.9–10.1
Alanine aminotransaminase, U/L	1,599	7–45
Aspartate aminotransaminase, U/L	700	8–48
Alkaline phosphatase, U/L	294	45–115
Uric acid, mg/dL	14.4	3.7–8.0
Lactate, mmol/L	15	0.6–2.3
Hemoglobin, g/dL	10.0	13.5–17.5
Leukocytes, ×10^9/L	420	3.5–10.5
Blasts and promonocytes, %	77	<1
Platelets, ×10^9/L	263	150–450
Prothrombin time, s	41.4	9.5–13.8
International normalized ratio	3.7	0.8–1.2
Partial thromboplastin time, s	51	28–38
Fibrinogen, mg/dL	<60	200–375

bicarbonate 12 mmol/L. A chest radiograph showed bilateral perihilar infiltrates and pleural effusions.

The patient's presentation was concerning for leukostasis with acute myeloid leukemia (AML) complicated by disseminated intravascular coagulation (DIC) and spontaneous tumor lysis syndrome (TLS). Fresh frozen plasma and cryoprecipitate were administered to facilitate placement of a double-lumen dialysis catheter to begin leukapheresis. Soon after its placement, however, the patient had an asystolic cardiac arrest and could not be resuscitated.

DISCUSSION

The term *hyperleukocytosis* is generally used to define a total leukocyte count greater than 100×10^9/L or a blast cell count greater than 50×10^9/L.

Hyperleukocytosis with concurrent symptoms of hyperviscosity or impaired tissue perfusion is termed *leukostasis*, which is an oncologic emergency. Leukostasis occurs most typically in a blast crisis associated with AML or chronic myeloid leukemia (CML).

Leukostasis, which may be the presenting feature of AML in 5% to 18% of patients, is associated with a mortality rate of up to 30%, especially among elderly patients with poor performance status, coagulopathy, respiratory compromise, and multiorgan dysfunction (1). Leukemic blasts possess high metabolic activity and produce various cytokines, in addition to expressing vascular endothelial adhesion molecules (2). They are less deformable than mature leukocytes and form plugs in the microcirculatory beds of various organs (2). These processes give rise to the clinical manifestations of leukostasis, such as visual disturbances, altered consciousness, intracranial hemorrhage, respiratory failure from noncardiogenic pulmonary edema, and acute kidney injury (1). The patient described above presented with most of these typical manifestations, although brain imaging would have been useful to rule out intracranial hemorrhage.

In patients with AML or CML, leukocyte counts greater than 100×10^9/L put patients at an increased risk for leukostasis, but in patients with acute or chronic lymphoblastic leukemias, leukocyte counts as high as 400×10^9/L may not cause leukostasis. This difference has been attributed to the smaller size, decreased endothelial adherence, and higher deformability of lymphoblasts compared to myeloid precursors (1).

Laboratory test results are often misleading in leukostasis, so they must be interpreted with great caution. Fragments of leukemic blasts can be mislabeled as platelets by automated counters, thus causing overestimation of the platelet count (3). Potassium levels may also be overestimated in leukostasis and may result from in vitro lysis of blast cells or release of intracellular potassium during transport in pneumatic tube systems (4). Blood samples should be carried relatively undisturbed to the laboratory and analyzed immediately or tested at the point of care. The Pao_2 may be spuriously low because of oxygen consumption by the highly metabolic leukemic blasts, and fingertip pulse oximetry provides a more accurate estimation of oxygen content of blood in patients with leukostasis (5). As in the patient described above, DIC and spontaneous TLS may coexist with leukostasis, so appropriate laboratory investigations to confirm these diagnoses should be performed.

As stated above, leukostasis is an oncologic emergency, and treatment should proceed expeditiously. Aggressive intravascular hydration should be initiated and a hematologist must be consulted early. Leukapheresis can be initiated quickly and leads to prompt leukoreduction, but leukapheresis does not address the primary pathology in the bone marrow, so induction chemotherapy should be initiated as soon as possible. Hydroxyurea is also used at dosages of 20 to 30 mg/kg daily or higher to achieve leukoreduction, but this agent does not take effect for at least 1 to 2 days (1). Allopurinol is usually given before chemotherapy for TLS prophylaxis. Red blood cell transfusions should be avoided in the acute phase to prevent worsening hyperviscosity, and leukapheresis should be avoided in patients with acute promyelocytic leukemia (French-American-British classification M3) because of the risk of exacerbating acute DIC (1).

REFERENCES

1. Wieduwilt MJ, Damon LE. Critical care of patients with hematologic malignancies. In: Irwin RS, Rippe JM, eds. Irwin and Rippe's intensive care medicine. 7th ed. Philadelphia (PA): Wolters Kluwer Health/Lippincott Williams & Wilkins; c2012. p. 1284–96.

2. Stucki A, Rivier AS, Gikic M, Monai N, Schapira M, Spertini O. Endothelial cell activation by myeloblasts: molecular mechanisms of leukostasis and leukemic cell dissemination. Blood. 2001 Apr 1;97(7):2121–9.

3. Hammerstrom J. Spurious platelet counts in acute leukaemia with DIC due to cell fragmentation. Clin Lab Haematol. 1992;14(3):239–43.

4. Garwicz D, Karlman M. Early recognition of reverse pseudohyperkalemia in heparin plasma samples during leukemic hyperleukocytosis can prevent iatrogenic hypokalemia. Clin Biochem. 2012 Dec;45(18):1700–2. Epub 2012 Aug 1.

5. Gorski TF, Ajemian M, Hussain E, Talhouk A, Ruskin G, Hanna A, et al Correlation of pseudohypoxemia and leukocytosis in chronic lymphocytic leukemia. South Med J. 1999 Aug;92(8):817–9.

Reverse Apical Ballooning Syndrome Due to Clonidine Withdrawal

PRAMOD K. GURU, MBBS,
DEREDDI RAJA S. REDDY, MD,
AND NANDAN S. ANAVEKAR, MB, BCH

CASE PRESENTATION

A 59-year-old white woman presented with shortness of breath and subacute, nonradiating chest pain. She had no known history of coronary artery disease or hypertension, but she did have a remote history of pulmonary thromboembolism along with chronic obstructive pulmonary disease, hypothyroidism, and chronic low back pain. For her chronic back pain, she had been treated with an intrathecal pump containing a mixture of fentanyl, hydromorphone, bupivacaine, and clonidine for the past 14 years.

On the day before the patient's admission, clonidine had been discontinued for unclear reasons. When she arrived at the hospital, her blood pressure was 190/100 mm Hg, but the other clinical examination findings were unremarkable. The initial electrocardiogram showed ST-segment depression and T-wave inversion in the inferior chest wall and lateral precordial leads. Initial levels of troponin I and the N-terminal fragment of the precursor to B-type natriuretic peptide (NT-proBNP) were significantly elevated. Results were normal for other laboratory tests, including those for hemoglobin, electrolytes, and liver and kidney function. Given her history of smoking and prior episode of venous thromboembolism, initial diagnostic considerations included acute coronary syndrome and recurrent pulmonary embolism. Urgently performed transthoracic echocardiography showed significant regional wall motion abnormalities. The mid-basal ventricle was dilated and akinetic, whereas the apex was hypercontractile. Overall, the left ventricular ejection fraction was estimated to be around 25%. The patient was admitted to the coronary care unit and underwent contrast-enhanced cardiac computed tomography (CT) that showed an absence of pulmonary embolism, normal aortic anatomy, mild coronary artery disease, and biventricular dysfunction with basal and midventricular segmental akinesis and apical hyperkinesis (Figure 17.1). She then underwent coronary angiography that showed a left-dominant circulation with no significant coronary artery disease.

A diagnosis of reverse apical ballooning syndrome due to clonidine withdrawal was based on the findings from echocardiography, CT of the chest, and coronary angiography. Clonidine withdrawal was thought to be the most likely explanation for the accelerated hypertension and cardiac dysfunction because of the recent abrupt discontinuation of clonidine along with the absence of other precipitating factors.

After angiography, oral clonidine was reinstituted along with β-blockers. The patient's blood pressure improved considerably, and she had no further episodes of chest pain. Oral clonidine was tapered and stopped while she was in the hospital. She was discharged with a β-blocker and an angiotensin-converting enzyme inhibitor. Follow-up transthoracic echocardiography at 6 weeks showed resolution

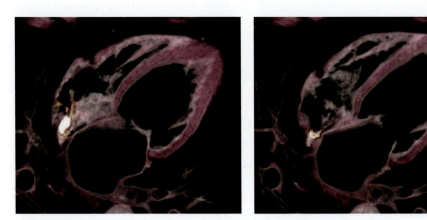

FIGURE 17.1. Cardiac Computed Tomographic Imaging. Apical systolic contraction is preserved, but basal contraction is absent. Left, Systole. Right, Diastole.

of the regional wall motion abnormalities with normalization of left ventricular function and a left ventricular ejection fraction of 64%.

DISCUSSION

Apical ballooning syndrome, also known as stress cardiomyopathy or takotsubo cardiomyopathy, is a reversible condition that mimics acute coronary syndrome (1). Takotsubo cardiomyopathy, first described in Japan in the early 1990s, was named after *tako tsubo*, which means octopus pot or trap in Japanese, because the characteristic hyperkinetic basal and akinetic and bulging apical segments that are typically seen in this disorder resemble an octopus trap. Most of the early reported cases occurred in postmenopausal women in association with acute, stressful situations. The unique pathophysiologic feature is the transient apical systolic dysfunction of the left ventricle without any structural coronary artery abnormality. Over the past several years, case reports of variant takotsubo cardiomyopathy have been described in which the regional wall motion abnormalities do not resemble the original description of this syndrome (2). Reverse apical ballooning syndrome is an infrequently described variant, in which contractility of the apical segments is preserved but the mid and basal segments are dysfunctional. The occurrence of both typical and variant takotsubo cardiomyopathy is increasingly recognized in critical care medicine.

Reverse apical ballooning syndrome in association with clonidine withdrawal has not been previously described in the medical literature. Ennezat et al (2) coined the term *inverted takotsubo* to describe the syndrome in patients with acute cerebral disorders. Subsequently, in 2006, Hurst et al (3) reported a case series of 4 patients who had midventricular ballooning related to vigorous exercise, severe anxiety, and postoperative status. The exact prevalence of the condition is not known, although the incidence of stress cardiomyopathy in the United States has been reported to be as high as 34,000 cases per year (4,5). The variants of takotsubo cardiomyopathy described in the literature consist of akinesis or dyskinesis of the mid and basal segments, akinesis or dyskinesis of the anterolateral or posterior basal segments, and midventricular and right ventricular dysfunction (1,3,5).

The pathophysiology of either classic or variant takotsubo cardiomyopathy is not clearly understood. The most consistent and widely accepted theory is that exaggerated sympathetic stimulation leads to catecholamine-induced cardiotoxicity (5). The other postulated mechanisms involve coronary thrombosis, abnormal vasoreactivity, and impaired fatty acid metabolism. The variations in the wall motion abnormality have been attributed to regional differences and individual variations in adrenergic sensitivity or innervation (or both) (1). The characteristic findings of takotsubo cardiomyopathy on histopathology are diffuse inflammation and myocardial edema.

Clonidine is a pharmacologic agent that has been used primarily in the management of hypertension, but it has also been used for pain management. It is a postganglionic α-agonist that acts mainly by reducing central sympathetic drive. Abruptly discontinued use of clonidine can lead to sudden sympathetic surges and clonidine withdrawal syndrome. The common manifestations of clonidine withdrawal are tachycardia and accelerated hypertension. Clinically, patients can present with chest pain, shortness of breath, hypotension or hypertension, and tachycardia mimicking an acute coronary syndrome. Patients can present with cardiogenic shock or with isolated cardiac enzyme elevations. Serial cardiac enzymes, urine catecholamine studies, viral serologies, CT of the chest, and coronary angiography have been advocated to exclude potentially life-threating conditions, such as acute coronary syndrome, pulmonary embolism, myocarditis, or aortic dissection.

Cardiac biomarkers are usually mildly elevated but are typically disproportionately low compared to the extent of ventricular dysfunction. The electrocardiogram is highly variable: It can be normal, or it can show significant ST-segment changes (including elevation or depression) along with associated T-wave abnormalities. The most characteristic finding is the absence of obstructive epicardial coronary artery disease at angiography along with the presence of severe regional wall motion abnormalities that do not correspond to any single coronary artery distribution territory. Both classic apical ballooning syndrome and its variants are characterized by an association with known triggering factors, minor electrocardiographic changes, minimal elevation of cardiac enzymes, and rapid recovery.

Reverse apical ballooning syndrome has also been reported in association with pheochromocytoma, serotonin syndrome, status epilepticus, status asthmaticus, pancreatitis, delirium tremens, subarachnoid hemorrhage, Guillain-Barré syndrome, cocaine use, septic shock, and administration of vasopressors (1,3–5). All these clinical entities are very common in intensive care unit patients and often carry a dismal prognosis. However, as the name suggests, stress cardiomyopathy is a reversible condition—if the trigger factor is removed and patients are adequately supported during the acute crisis. Most patients recover in 6 to 12 weeks after the event, with complete normalization of ventricular function (3,4).

In summary, awareness of the features of classic takotsubo cardiomyopathy and its variants can be helpful in managing these difficult clinical situations. The features include the echocardiographic findings, associated syndromes, and mild elevation of biomarkers.

ACKNOWLEDGMENT

Previously published in abstract form as Guru P, Vaidya V, Bierle D, Tajouri T, Anavekar N. Reverse apical ballooning syndrome: due to clonidine withdrawal [abstract]. Crit Care Med. 2013 Dec:41(12 Suppl); A297-8. Used with permission.

REFERENCES

1. Akashi YJ, Goldstein DS, Barbaro G, Ueyama T. Takotsubo cardiomyopathy: a new form of acute, reversible heart failure. Circulation. 2008 Dec 16;118(25):2754–62.

2. Ennezat PV, Pesenti-Rossi D, Aubert JM, Rachenne V, Bauchart JJ, Auffray JL, et al. Transient left ventricular basal dysfunction without coronary stenosis in acute cerebral disorders: a novel heart syndrome (inverted Takotsubo). Echocardiography. 2005 Aug;22(7):599–602.

3. Hurst RT, Askew JW, Reuss CS, Lee RW, Sweeney JP, Fortuin FD, et al. Transient midventricular ballooning syndrome: a new variant. J Am Coll Cardiol. 2006 Aug 1;48(3):579–83. Epub 2006 Jun 19.

4. Van de Walle SO, Gevaert SA, Gheeraert PJ, De Pauw M, Gillebert TC. Transient stress-induced cardiomyopathy with an "inverted takotsubo" contractile pattern. Mayo Clin Proc. 2006 Nov;81(11):1499–502.

5. Deshmukh A, Kumar G, Pant S, Rihal C, Murugiah K, Mehta JL. Prevalence of Takotsubo cardiomyopathy in the United States. Am Heart J. 2012 Jul;164(1):66–71. e1. Epub 2012 Jun 13.

A Well-Known Cardiac Condition With a Unique Presentation

SUMEDH S. HOSKOTE, MBBS,
MUHAMMAD A. RISHI, MBBS,
AND NATHAN J. SMISCHNEY, MD

CASE PRESENTATION

A 48-year-old woman with metastatic non–small cell lung cancer, associated meningeal carcinomatosis, recurrent partial seizures controlled with levetiracetam, and malignant pericardial effusion presented to the emergency department with left-sided hemiparesis. She had undergone pericardiocentesis 2 years earlier. Magnetic resonance imaging of the brain showed an acute infarct in the right cerebral hemisphere consistent with her symptoms. After admission to the general medical unit, she was noted to have right lower extremity edema, and duplex ultrasonography confirmed acute popliteal vein thrombosis. An unfractionated heparin infusion was started. Three days after heparin was started, she suddenly became tachycardic and dyspneic with labored respirations. Vital signs were notable for the following: heart rate 150 beats per minute, respirations 32 breaths per minute, blood pressure 150/100 mm Hg, and oxygen saturation 95% with oxygen delivered at 2 L/min through a nasal cannula. A 12-lead electrocardiogram showed sinus tachycardia at 150 beats per minute with right-axis deviation. Posteroanterior and lateral chest radiographs showed left lower lobe consolidation, likely loculated left pleural effusion, an enlarged cardiac silhouette,

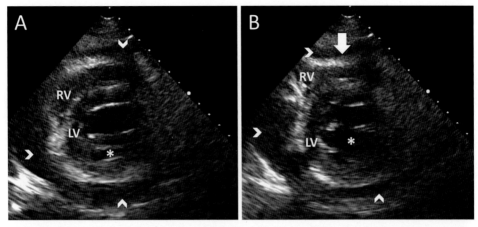

FIGURE 18.1. Transthoracic Echocardiogram, Parasternal Short-Axis View. A, Ventricular systole. B, Ventricular diastole. The asterisks indicate the mitral valve orifice, which is closed in systole (A) and open in diastole (B). The arrowheads indicate hypoechoic material surrounding the heart, consistent with a pericardial effusion. The arrow indicates a concave indentation in the right ventricular (RV) wall during diastole (B), which is consistent with cardiac tamponade. LV indicates left ventricle.

and pulmonary vascular congestion. The patient was transferred to the medical intensive care unit for further management.

A bedside ultrasonographic examination of the thorax showed pericardial effusion and left pleural effusion. A formal transthoracic echocardiogram (TTE) not only confirmed the pleural and pericardial effusions but also showed complete right atrial and right ventricular diastolic collapse consistent with cardiac tamponade (Figure 18.1). With pericardiocentesis, 450 mL of serosanguineous pericardial fluid was evacuated, and the patient's hemodynamic status stabilized. A pericardial drain was placed for continued drainage in case of reaccumulation. The left-sided pleural effusion was also drained. Both effusions were positive for malignant cells. The patient improved and was discharged to the general medical unit to receive palliative care.

DISCUSSION

The classic triad of low arterial blood pressure, distended neck veins, and muffled heart sounds is known as the Beck triad and is associated with cardiac tamponade. The full triad, however, is quite uncommon in cases of tamponade, and the diagnosis requires a high degree of awareness. Atypical presentations of cardiac tamponade can be diagnosed earlier with the use of bedside cardiac ultrasonography, which is now commonplace in the intensive care unit.

Cardiac tamponade can occur when intrapericardial pressure exceeds the diastolic pressure in the cardiac chambers (1). It can occur with a pericardial effusion of any size and progress to cardiac arrest unless it is diagnosed and treated promptly. Tamponade is generally thought of as being linked to hypotension; however, hypotension is present in only 26% of patients with cardiac tamponade (2). Some patients with tamponade may present with elevated blood pressure from underlying hypertension or high adrenergic tone (3), which was likely present in the patient described above. Muffled heart sounds are only 28% sensitive for tamponade (2). More reliable physical findings include pulsus paradoxus of 12 mm Hg or more (sensitivity 98%, specificity 83%) and tachycardia, tachypnea, and elevated jugular venous pressure (sensitivities 76%-82%) (2). Many patients may not have the electrocardiographic parameters considered typical of pericardial effusion or tamponade, such as low QRS voltage (sensitivity 10%, specificity 98%), PR-segment depression (sensitivity 28%, specificity 87%), and electrical alternans (sensitivity 3%, specificity 92%) (4).

Cardiac tamponade is often a clinical diagnosis when the appropriate clinical context and typical clinical features are present. However, subtle or atypical clinical and electrocardiographic findings are sometimes present, which may delay the clinical diagnosis of cardiac tamponade. TTE must be performed if a patient is suspected of having pericardial effusion or if a patient with pericarditis or pericardial effusion presents with clinical deterioration. In the case presented above, bedside TTE was vital in rapidly identifying the cause of the patient's deterioration. Intensivists must be familiar with echocardiographic findings associated with tamponade in order to make a prompt diagnosis before a formal TTE can be performed.

Initially, increased intrapericardial pressure compresses the low-pressure atria, especially in diastole. A progressive increase in intrapericardial pressure leads to compression of the right ventricle, which leads to compromised cardiac output (1). The earliest echocardiographic sign of cardiac tamponade is atrial diastolic collapse; however, this finding alone is not very specific (1). Right atrial collapse, especially when it persists for more than one-third of the cardiac cycle, is highly sensitive and specific for cardiac tamponade (5). Left atrial collapse is seen in only 25% of patients with tamponade but is highly specific when present (5). Right ventricular diastolic collapse is more significant and more specific for tamponade (1). The inferior vena cava is usually dilated with decreased inspiratory collapse due to impaired cardiac filling (5).

REFERENCES

1. Pericardial disease. In: Ryding A. Essential echocardiography. 2nd ed. Edinburgh (Scotland): Churchill Livingstone/Elsevier; c2013. p. 180–91.

2. Fang JC, O'Gara PT. The history and physical examination: an evidence-based approach. In: Bonow RO, Mann DL, Zipes DP, Libby P, editors. Braunwald's heart disease: a textbook of cardiovascular medicine. 9th ed. Philadelphia (PA): Saunders/Elsevier; c2012. p. 107–25.

3. Spodick DH. Acute cardiac tamponade. N Engl J Med. 2003 Aug 14;349(7):684–90.

4. Eisenberg MJ, de Romeral LM, Heidenreich PA, Schiller NB, Evans GT Jr. The diagnosis of pericardial effusion and cardiac tamponade by 12-lead ECG: a technology assessment. Chest. 1996 Aug;110(2):318–24.

5. Hoit BD. Pericardial disease and pericardial tamponade. Crit Care Med. 2007 Aug;35(8 Suppl):S355–64.

Electrolyte Abnormalities During Continuous Renal Replacement Therapy

SUMEDH S. HOSKOTE, MBBS,
FOUAD T. CHEBIB, MD,
AND NATHAN J. SMISCHNEY, MD

CASE PRESENTATION

A 26-year-old woman with a history of orthotopic heart transplant for Ebstein anomaly was admitted with cardiogenic shock secondary to graft vasculopathy. She was treated with antithymocyte globulin, high-dose methylprednisolone, azathioprine, mycophenolate mofetil, and tacrolimus; however, her cardiac function did not recover appreciably. Despite treatment with several vasoactive agents, she had refractory hypotension. She was taken to the operating room for initiation of venoarterial extracorporeal membrane oxygenation as a bridge to mechanical cardiac support or transplant. As a consequence of the cardiogenic shock and intraoperative hypotension, anuric acute kidney injury (Acute Kidney Injury Network stage 3) developed, with the creatinine level peaking at 2.7 mg/dL. The patient required initiation of continuous renal replacement therapy (CRRT) for fluid and electrolyte management. She received broad coverage with antimicrobials, including vancomycin, piperacillin-tazobactam, and caspofungin, in addition to *Pneumocystis jiroveci* prophylaxis with sulfamethoxazole-trimethoprim. Total parenteral nutrition had been initiated 2 days earlier. Her CRRT settings are shown in Table 19.1. Notable results from her most recent blood tests are shown in Table 19.2.

The laboratory data showed a total calcium to ionized calcium ratio of 2.8 with an elevated anion gap suggestive of citrate accumulation. After the citrate infusion was decreased to 250 mL hourly, laboratory test results were total calcium 10.2 mg/dL and ionized calcium 4.7 mg/dL, which indicated resolution of citrate toxicity.

TABLE 19.1. Settings for Continuous Renal Replacement Therapy

Component	Setting
Total hemofiltration rate (at 30 mL/kg hourly), mL/h	3,000
Blood flow rate, mL/min	200
Anticoagulant citrate dextrose solution, solution A (ACD-A), mL/h	300
Calcium chloride, g daily	22
Sodium phosphate, mmol daily	85
Replacement fluid (50% given prefilter; 50% given postfilter)	
Bicarbonate, mmol/L	22
Potassium, mmol/L	4

TABLE 19.2. Latest Blood Test Results

Component	Value	Reference Range
Sodium, mmol/L	137	135–145
Chloride, mmol/L	103	100–108
Potassium, mmol/L	4.5	3.6–5.2
Bicarbonate, mmol/L	18	22–29
Serum urea nitrogen, mg/dL	9	6–21
Creatinine, mg/dL	<0.4	0.7–1.2
Calcium (total), mg/dL	11.2	8.9–10.0
Calcium (ionized), mg/dL	4.02	4.65–5.30
Magnesium, mg/dL	1.7	1.7–203
Inorganic phosphorous, mg/dL	3.3	2.5–4.5
Albumin, g/dL	2.6	3.5–5.0
Total bilirubin, mg/dL	13.8	0.1–1.0
Direct bilirubin, mg/dL	11.0	0.0–0.3
Alanine transaminase, U/L	524	7–45
Prothrombin time, s	13.6	9.5–13.8

DISCUSSION

CRRT is increasingly used in the management of acute kidney injury in critically ill patients (1). Given the relatively slow fluid and solute removal, CRRT may offer better hemodynamic stability when compared to intermittent hemodialysis. Regional citrate anticoagulation is currently recommended by the Kidney Disease: Improving Global Outcomes consensus group as the preferred anticoagulant for CRRT in patients with or without increased bleeding risk (levels of evidence 2B and 2C, respectively) (1). Although well-tolerated in general, CRRT may cause serious and life-threatening electrolyte imbalances that require urgent intervention by the intensivist.

Citrate is used in CRRT as a regional anticoagulant. Infused into the afferent blood line, citrate chelates ionized calcium, thereby preventing the progression of the coagulation cascade. The majority of the calcium citrate complex is removed across the hemofilter, and the remainder is metabolized by the liver, kidney, and skeletal muscle. Each citrate molecule potentially produces 3 bicarbonate molecules through metabolism in the Krebs cycle (2). Calcium released from the calcium citrate complex, along with a continuous calcium infusion, restores serum ionized calcium concentrations. Normalization of serum ionized calcium levels by these means restricts the anticoagulant action of citrate to the CRRT hemofilter and tubing, where ionized calcium levels may be less than 2 mg/dL.

Citrate toxicity may occur in patients receiving CRRT who have reduced citrate metabolism, particularly those with liver failure. An increase in the total calcium level accompanied by a decrease in ionized calcium that results in a ratio of total calcium to ionized calcium of 2.5 or higher may indicate citrate toxicity (3,4). The presence of a high anion gap metabolic acidosis usually indicates hypercitratemia with low serum bicarbonate in this clinical setting. The patient described above was receiving parenteral nutrition, caspofungin, piperacillin-tazobactam, and sulfamethoxazole-trimethoprim, and congestive or ischemic liver injury probably occurred secondary to cardiogenic shock, all of which are associated with liver injury that is hepatocellular or cholestatic or both. Impaired hepatic function in this patient likely resulted in citrate accumulation, which led to various biochemical abnormalities. When citrate toxicity is suspected, the rate of citrate infusion should be decreased, and laboratory tests must be rechecked regularly to ensure resolution of the toxicity. Further adjustments to the calcium infusion may be required depending on electrolyte results. Decreasing the citrate dose may increase the likelihood of recurrent hemofilter clotting. This may be managed by 1) decreasing the filtration fraction by increasing the blood flow rate or decreasing the ultrafiltration rate or 2) increasing the prefilter replacement fluid fraction to dilute the blood going through the filter and decrease the risk of filter clotting.

Aside from citrate toxicity, several other biochemical abnormalities may occur in patients receiving CRRT, so it is imperative to frequently monitor serum electrolytes, total and ionized calcium, and acid-base balance (5). These biochemical abnormalities include the following:

- Hypophosphatemia, hypokalemia, and hypomagnesemia may occur during CRRT if replacement of these electrolytes is inadequate. Treatment is enteral or parenteral replacement as needed.
- Hypocalcemia, associated with decreased total and ionized calcium levels, can also occur in the absence of citrate toxicity if calcium replacement is inadequate.
- Hypercalcemia, associated with elevations of both total and ionized calcium levels, may occur with excessive calcium replacement.
- Hypernatremia due to use of trisodium citrate anticoagulation may occur if the sodium concentration in the replacement fluid is not decreased.
- Metabolic alkalosis due to the use of citrate anticoagulation can occur if the bicarbonate level in the replacement fluid is not adequately decreased (citrate metabolism in the liver itself produces bicarbonate).

REFERENCES

1. Hoste EA, Dhondt A. Clinical review: use of renal replacement therapies in special groups of ICU patients. Crit Care. 2012 Jan 19;16(1):201.

2. Davenport A, Tolwani A. Citrate anticoagulation for continuous renal replacement therapy (CRRT) in patients with acute kidney injury admitted to the intensive care unit. NDT Plus. 2009;2(6):439-47.

3. Schultheiss C, Saugel B, Phillip V, Thies P, Noe S, Mayr U, et al. Continuous venovenous hemodialysis with regional citrate anticoagulation in patients with liver failure: a prospective observational study. Crit Care. 2012 Aug 22;16(4):R162.

4. Link A, Klingele M, Speer T, Rbah R, Poss J, Lerner-Graber A, et al. Total-to-ionized calcium ratio predicts mortality in continuous renal replacement therapy with citrate anticoagulation in critically ill patients. Crit Care. 2012 May 29;16(3):R97.

5. Fall P, Szerlip HM. Continuous renal replacement therapy: cause and treatment of electrolyte complications. Semin Dial. 2010 Nov-Dec;23(6):581-5. Epub 2010 Dec 20.

A Disease Masquerading as Septic Shock

MUHAMMAD A. RISHI, MBBS, AND NATHAN J. SMISCHNEY, MD

CASE PRESENTATION

An 82-year-old man presented with a severe headache, a several-day history of nausea and vomiting, and hypotension. He had a past medical history significant for saddle pulmonary embolism (he was receiving warfarin for anticoagulation), congestive heart failure, type 2 diabetes mellitus, hypertension, degenerative joint disease, and monoclonal gammopathy of undetermined significance. He was admitted to the intensive care unit.

The patient was initially treated with intravenous fluids for volume resuscitation and broad-spectrum antibiotics (ampicillin, vancomycin, and ceftriaxone) because of concerns of possible meningitis. Findings were unremarkable from blood and cerebrospinal fluid cultures and a chest radiograph. Urine culture grew *Enterococcus*. Computed tomography (CT) of the head was negative for hemorrhage and acute ischemia. The patient's symptoms rapidly improved over the next 24 hours. His antibiotic therapy was narrowed to only vancomycin, and he was transferred to the general medicine unit.

Shortly after being transferred, the patient became hypotensive with altered mental status, fever, and tachycardia, prompting immediate fluid resuscitation and transfer back to the intensive care unit. Broad-spectrum antibiotics (ampicillin, vancomycin, ceftriaxone, and levofloxacin) were administered along with acyclovir, and he underwent volume resuscitation, resulting in an improvement in his

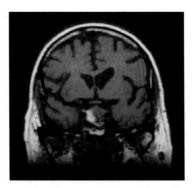

FIGURE 20.1. Pituitary Apoplexy. Noncontrast magnetic resonance image shows a T1-hyperintense mass within the sella that is consistent with subacute pituitary hemorrhage.

blood pressure and urine output. Renal ultrasonographic findings were normal, with no evidence of hydronephrosis. Laboratory test results included low serum cortisol, low free thyroxine, low thyrotropin, and hypernatremia. These findings, along with increased urine output, made a diagnosis of pituitary apoplexy more likely, and the patient was given high-dose hydrocortisone, desmopressin acetate, and fludrocortisone. Noncontrast magnetic resonance imaging (MRI) of the head showed a T1-hyperintense mass within the sella that was consistent with subacute pituitary hemorrhage (Figure 20.1). With hormone replacement, the patient's hemodynamic status dramatically improved, his mentation cleared, and he was transferred back to the general medical unit.

DISCUSSION

Apoplexy of the pituitary gland is a clinical diagnosis and does not require pathologic confirmation (1). In different case series, the incidence ranges from 0.6% to 10%. Pituitary apoplexy is usually caused by hemorrhage, hemorrhagic infarction, or bland infarction of a pituitary adenoma. Peculiar vascularity of the pituitary gland and structural problems in small blood vessels in the suprasellar region may increase the risk of pituitary apoplexy. Pituitary apoplexy can be an elusive diagnosis because of its rarity and because pituitary adenoma can be undiagnosed at presentation (2).

The first symptom of pituitary apoplexy is usually severe, postorbital, frontal, or occipital headache. Headache is the most consistently described and the most frequently occurring symptom in patients with pituitary apoplexy. Nausea and vomiting are often severe. Diplopia and other cranial nerve palsies can be caused by lateral compression of the cavernous sinus contents. Similarly, superior sellar

A Respiratory Infection

KELLY A. CAWCUTT, MD,
AND CASSIE C. KENNEDY, MD

CASE PRESENTATION

A 74-year-old man with a past medical history significant for coronary artery disease, congestive heart failure with a left ventricular ejection fraction of 39%, asthma, and diabetes mellitus was admitted after 3 days of fever, fatigue, shortness of breath, and worsening cough with sputum production. The day before admission he was seen in an urgent care facility, where he was noted to have a stable cardiopulmonary status, although he had a cough and coarse breath sounds on examination. He was prescribed azithromycin and an albuterol inhaler with a plan for reevaluation if the symptoms worsened. No other testing was performed during that visit.

The patient's condition continued to worsen over the next 24 hours, and he presented to the emergency department the following day. Chest radiography did not show pulmonary infiltrates. Bacterial cultures were started and a nasopharyngeal swab for influenza testing was obtained. The CURB-65 (confusion, urea nitrogen, respiratory rate, blood pressure, age ≥65 years) score in the emergency department was 3, indicating severe risk with a predicted 30-day mortality of 14%. The patient was given an empirical dose of oseltamivir and admitted to the general medical unit. During the evening, he required intravenous fluid boluses for hypotension.

The following morning, his respiratory status continued to deteriorate, with increasing tachypnea and increased oxygen requirements. Arterial blood gas measurements showed severe acidemia (pH <7.0) with hypercapnia and hypoxia. The rapid response team was called, and he was transferred emergently to the medical intensive care unit (ICU) and intubated. Point-of-care ultrasonography showed no evidence of pneumothorax or deep vein thrombosis; a normal-sized, collapsible inferior vena cava with a decreased ejection fraction of 25% to 30%; and a small right ventricle. Formal venous ultrasonography and transthoracic echocardiography confirmed these findings. Chest radiography showed patchy opacities in the right mid and upper lung and in the left lung base that were more consistent with an infectious process than with pulmonary edema. For presumed septic shock and an elevated level of lactate, early goal-directed therapy was initiated with vasopressors and broad-spectrum antibiotics (vancomycin, levofloxacin, cefepime, metronidazole, and trimethoprim-sulfamethoxazole) in combination with the ongoing oseltamivir. Bronchoscopy was notable for erythematous mucosa throughout the bronchial tree, with minimal secretions but a progressively hemorrhagic return during bronchoalveolar lavage (BAL) that was suspicious for alveolar hemorrhage. The BAL fluid was submitted for microbiology testing.

Evaluation of the nasopharyngeal swab and the BAL fluid was positive for influenza A virus, and no other viral or bacterial microbiology results were positive. However, the patient had cardiac arrhythmias and died in the ICU.

This patient had received an annual influenza vaccination, but the vaccine efficacy varies for several reasons, including the overall match between the vaccine and the circulating virus, antigenic drift, and the recipient's immune response and age. The vaccine's efficacy is decreased in older patients. During the 2011-2012 influenza season, the overall (adjusted) vaccine efficacy was only 47% in preventing influenza that required medical attention. As a result of this variance, influenza may still develop in patients who have received the vaccine (1).

DISCUSSION

Influenza results from 3 species of RNA viruses that cause clinical illness: influenza A virus, influenza B virus, and influenza C virus. Influenza C virus causes a mild illness that does not require treatment and is therefore rarely discussed as being clinically relevant. Influenza A virus and influenza B virus form the seasonal influenza strains that are the focus of the guidelines for prevention, diagnosis, and treatment of influenza. Every year, on average, 5% to 20% of the US population is infected with influenza, which causes significant morbidity and mortality despite vaccination and the self-limited nature of most cases. In 2009, the H1N1 virus, an antigenic variant of *Influenzavirus A*, caused a pandemic that resulted in increased use of ICUs for patients with acute respiratory distress syndrome (ARDS). In the United States, 25% of hospitalized patients with H1N1 virus infection were admitted to an ICU, 63% required mechanical ventilation, 36% had ARDS, and 31% received a diagnosis of sepsis, with a death rate of 7%. The increase in critical care use during the 2009 pandemic heralded a renewed interest in management of severe influenza.

Influenza is an acute, febrile respiratory syndrome with potentially critical complications, including pneumonitis with hypoxemia, secondary bacterial pneumonia, ARDS, infectious alveolar hemorrhage, and septic shock with multiorgan failure. Risk factors for severe disease include the following: age younger than 2 years or older than 65 years, American Indian or Alaskan native ethnicity, chronic cardiopulmonary disease, diabetes mellitus, immunosuppression, pregnancy or within 2 weeks post partum, and morbid obesity.

During influenza season, all patients admitted to the ICU with fever and respiratory symptoms should be tested for influenza. Elderly patients who present initially with fever but no respiratory symptoms should also be tested. Diagnostic influenza testing should be performed as soon as possible, ideally within 5 days after symptom onset. Nasopharyngeal swabs or aspirates are usually preferred for adults, but for patients who are undergoing mechanical ventilation, upper and lower respiratory tract samples (from endotracheal aspiration or BAL) should be evaluated (2).

Hospitalized patients should receive antiviral therapy for suspected or confirmed influenza, preferably with oseltamivir, zanamivir, or peramivir, even if more than 48 hours has passed since symptom onset. Respiratory droplet precautions should be instituted for all these patients. In the 2009 pandemic, oseltamivir-resistant strains of the H1N1 virus were documented; however, the prevalence remains low (3). In the 2009 pandemic, critically ill patients who had limited gastric absorption (eg, septic shock with poor limited gut perfusion or gastrointestinal hemorrhage) were eligible for compassionate use of intravenous zanamivir, although its availability was limited. At publication, intravenous zanamivir was available only as an investigational drug through clinical trials; however, intravenous peramivir is available, but efficacy data on hospitalized patients are limited (4).

Additional therapies for critically ill patients with influenza also garnered much attention after the 2009 pandemic. Extracorporeal membrane oxygenation was used successfully for refractory hypoxemia in patients with ARDS from influenza. Corticosteroids should not be used because of the potential for prolonged viral replication and worse overall outcomes.

Additional therapies, such as monoclonal antibodies, convalescent plasma (5), and hyperimmune intravenous immunoglobulin, are not routinely recommended currently.

Even more than 48 hours after symptom onset, inpatients who have suspected or confirmed influenza should receive antiviral therapy, and respiratory droplet precautions should be instituted.

REFERENCES

1. Harper SA, Bradley JS, Englund JA, File TM, Gravenstein S, Hayden FG, et al; Expert Panel of the Infectious Diseases Society of America. Seasonal influenza in adults and children: diagnosis, treatment, chemoprophylaxis, and institutional outbreak management: clinical practice guidelines of the Infectious Diseases Society of America. Clin Infect Dis. 2009 Apr 15;48(8):1003–32.

2. Uyeki TM. Preventing and controlling influenza with available interventions. N Engl J Med. 2014 Feb 27;370(9):789–91. Epub 2014 Jan 22.

3. Harter G, Zimmermann O, Maier L, Schubert A, Mertens T, Kern P, et al. Intravenous zanamivir for patients with pneumonitis due to pandemic (H1N1) 2009 influenza virus. Clin Infect Dis. 2010 May 1;50(9):1249–51.

4. Leider JP, Brunker PA, Ness PM. Convalescent transfusion for pandemic influenza: preparing blood banks for a new plasma product? Transfusion. 2010 Jun;50(6):1384–98. Epub 2010 Feb 11.

5. Ohmit SE, Thompson MG, Petrie JG, Thaker SN, Jackson ML, Belongia EA, et al. Influenza vaccine effectiveness in the 2011-2012 season: protection against each circulating virus and the effect of prior vaccination on estimates. Clin Infect Dis. 2014 Feb;58(3):319–27. Epub 2013 Nov 13.

Infection in a Patient With Chronic Myeloid Leukemia

MICHELLE BIEHL, MD, LISBETH Y. GARCIA ARGUELLO, MD, AND TENG MOUA, MD

CASE PRESENTATION

A 31-year-old man with a medical history significant for chronic myeloid leukemia complicated by blast transformation was admitted 8 days after he received a matched unrelated donor hematopoietic stem cell transplant. He presented with severe generalized pain, intractable nausea, and right upper quadrant (RUQ) abdominal tenderness; he was afebrile and hemodynamically stable. Physical examination revealed a subcutaneous, pea-sized nodule without erythema or color change in the RUQ of the abdomen. On abdominal ultrasonography, a small amount of free fluid was identified adjacent to the liver and gallbladder in addition to gallbladder wall distention and the presence of biliary sludge. Prophylactic antibiotic therapy included penicillin V, levofloxacin, metronidazole, acyclovir, and caspofungin. Voriconazole was not given because the patient had a history of transaminitis.

On hospital day 3, the patient had a cough, mild hemoptysis, pleuritic chest pain, and an enlarging, firm, coin-sized ecchymotic subcutaneous nodule in the RUQ of the abdomen. Chest radiography showed right upper lobe alveolar infiltrate that was confirmed with computed tomography of the chest, which also showed acute pulmonary embolism in segmental and subsegmental right upper

lobe pulmonary arteries, multiple bilateral pulmonary nodules, mediastinal ade-
nopathy, and hypoattenuation within the spleen, which likely resulted from infarction. Duplex ultrasonography of the lower extremities was negative for thrombus.
Cefepime and vancomycin were added. A biopsy of the abdominal lesion was performed by a dermatologist.

The patient became hypotensive with respiratory distress, fever, and altered
mental status. He was transferred to the intensive care unit, where he was emergently intubated and mechanically ventilated on arrival. Bronchoscopy was performed, and bronchoalveolar lavage fluid was taken from the apical segment of the
right upper lobe. After a preliminary fungal smear showed an organism resembling
a fungus in the class Zygomycetes, intravenous amphotericin B liposomal complex
was added. Acrocyanosis was noted on the second and fourth fingers along with
circumferential purpuric contusions on the dorsum of the left hand; the abdominal lesion was becoming indurated and turning purplish. Subsequent computed
tomography of the abdomen and pelvis on hospital day 4 showed marked edema
and dilatation of the colon, with splenic and right renal infarcts. The skin biopsy
results showed angioinvasive hyphal elements consistent with Zygomycetes,
which confirmed the diagnosis of widely disseminated mucormycosis.

The patient's status continued to deteriorate, with persistent fever, hypoxemia,
multiple skin lesions, and severe neutropenia. He underwent another broncho-
scopic evaluation on hospital day 9, which showed multiple areas of luminal
obstruction from dried bloody casts and necrotic mucosa, most significantly at
the proximal left main bronchus near the carina. Despite aggressive efforts, the
patient's condition progressed to septic shock and severe acute respiratory distress syndrome. After the medical team had an extensive discussion with his family, the patient was transitioned to comfort care, and he died on hospital day 15.
Autopsy results showed widely disseminated zygomycosis with multiple hemorrhagic infarcts in the brain, lungs, spleen, gallbladder, kidneys, and skin.

DISCUSSION

Mucormycosis is a severe fungal infection that carries significant morbidity
and mortality, particularly in immunocompromised patients (1). It is the third
most common fungal infection after invasive aspergillosis and candidiasis (2).
The incidence of mucormycosis among patients who have had a hematopoietic stem cell transplant (HSCT) is 0.1% to 2.0%; patients with an allogeneic

HLA-unrelated donor transplant are at higher risk than those with an autologous transplant (3). Primary risk factors for mucormycosis in patients with HSCT include severe graft-versus-host disease, use of high-dose corticosteroids, previous cytomegalovirus or respiratory viral disease, older age, complicated diabetes mellitus, malnutrition, and use of voriconazole either prophylactically or therapeutically (1,4).

The main transmission route of Zygomycetes is airborne, but ingestion and direct skin inoculation are also possible. Angioinvasion is a hallmark of mucormycosis, leading to tissue infarction and necrosis (4). Symptoms vary depending on the affected organ. Disseminated disease may originate from any primary site: rhino-orbital-cerebral, pulmonary, gastrointestinal, cutaneous, renal, or the central nervous system (4).

A high level of awareness is required to diagnose mucormycosis. Biopsy with histopathologic confirmation of fungal invasion is the best diagnostic tool (Figure 22.1). It should show wide, ribbonlike, aseptate hyphae that branch at a 90° angle. Organisms are often surrounded by necrotic debris. *Aspergillus*

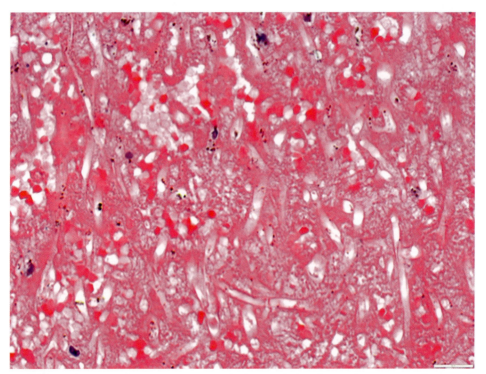

FIGURE 22.1. Mucormycosis. Histopathology of the lung shows an infarct with intravascular fungal organisms.

organisms may look similar; however, their septate hyphae are thinner and branch at a 45° angle. Zygomycetes organisms are rarely isolated from cultures of blood, cerebrospinal fluid, sputum, urine, feces, or swabs of infected areas (4). Although a sterile culture does not exclude infection (because the organism may be killed during tissue processing), a lone positive culture is not sufficient to establish a diagnosis of infection because the fungus is ubiquitous in nature and can colonize healthy persons and be considered a contaminant (4). Despite its fast rate of growth, Zygomycetes organisms may not grow in culture, so polymerase chain reaction testing may be an alternative (2); however, this tool still requires more investigation before it will be commonly used.

When mucormycosis is suspected, treatment should begin immediately, with aggressive débridement of infected and necrotic tissue and antifungal therapy. Amphotericin B liposomal complex is the preferred first-line agent. The prognosis for patients with disseminated mucormycosis, though, is very poor, even with aggressive therapy. Median survival of HSCT patients with mucormycosis is less than 2 months, with a mortality rate of 75% (1). In a large case series of 929 reported cases of mucormycosis, 100% of patients with disseminated disease died (5).

Disseminated mucormycosis is a devastating fungal infection causing significant morbidity and mortality. Recognizing it early in immunocompromised or at-risk patients is key. Biopsy is crucial because the diagnosis is defined by histopathologic detection of fungal elements in affected organs. Invasive disease requires prompt management with surgical débridement and antifungal therapy. Despite all efforts, morbidity and mortality are still high.

REFERENCES

1. Lanternier F, Sun HY, Ribaud P, Singh N, Kontoyiannis DP, Lortholary O. Mucormycosis in organ and stem cell transplant recipients. Clin Infect Dis. 2012 Jun;54(11):1629–36. Epub 2012 Mar 19.

2. Hammond SP, Bialek R, Milner DA, Petschnigg EM, Baden LR, Marty FM. Molecular methods to improve diagnosis and identification of mucormycosis. J Clin Microbiol. 2011 Jun;49(6):2151–3. Epub 2011 Apr 20.

3. Park BJ, Pappas PG, Wannemuehler KA, Alexander BD, Anaissie EJ, Andes DR, et al. Invasive non-Aspergillus mold infections in transplant recipients, United States, 2001-2006. Emerg Infect Dis. 2011 Oct;17(10):1855–64.

4. Spellberg B, Edwards J Jr, Ibrahim A. Novel perspectives on mucormycosis: pathophysiology, presentation, and management. Clin Microbiol Rev. 2005 Jul;18(3):556–69.

5. Roden MM, Zaoutis TE, Buchanan WL, Knudsen TA, Sarkisova TA, Schaufele RL, et al. Epidemiology and outcome of zygomycosis: a review of 929 reported cases. Clin Infect Dis. 2005 Sep 1;41(5):634–53. Epub 2005 Jul 29.

Torsades de Pointes

ANDREA B. JOHNSON, APRN, CNP,
AND THOMAS B. COMFERE, MD

CASE PRESENTATION

A 66-year-old man with a past medical history of mantle cell lymphoma was admitted to the hospital for neutropenic fever, nausea, and suspected periengraftment syndrome on day 16 after autologous stem cell transplant. He was treated with antibiotics, antiemetics, and corticosteroids and was recovering well. On the expected day of dismissal, he complained of some light-headedness and mild dyspnea, prompting a 12-lead electrocardiogram, which showed normal sinus rhythm with a corrected QT interval (QTc) of 526 ms. He was transferred to the intensive care unit for further management; shortly after arrival, an irregular rhythm developed with bigeminy and runs of nonsustained ventricular tachycardia, which ultimately degenerated to torsades de pointes without hemodynamic compromise.

Laboratory evaluation was significant for a potassium level of 3.5 mmol/L and a magnesium level of 1.8 mg/dL. Immediate interventions included 4 mg magnesium intravenously (IV) (before the laboratory test results were available), with a brief resolution of the torsades de pointes. However, an irregular baseline rhythm quickly returned, and the patient required further electrolyte replacement with magnesium and potassium.

β-Blockade was attempted with 2.5 mg of metoprolol IV, with a resultant worsening of the arrhythmia. Glycopyrrolate 0.4 mg IV was then administered in an attempt to suppress the arrhythmia by counteracting the negative chronotropic effect of the β-blockade by increasing the patient's heart rate and thereby shortening the QTc. This resulted in rapid improvement and a return to normal sinus rhythm. Over the next 24 hours, he received a total of 2 mg of glycopyrrolate in intermittent doses along with continued electrolyte replacement. Potentially offending pharmacologic agents, including prochlorperazine, were discontinued, and tight control of his electrolytes was maintained. He was eventually safely discharged from the hospital with no further documented cardiac events.

Further cardiovascular consultation with this patient identified a family history of a teenaged niece with sudden cardiac death. This prompted outpatient investigation into the possibility of a congenital component to his prolonged QTc. Genetic testing showed that he has genetically mediated type 2 long QT syndrome (LQTS). Options for his care include maximal β-blockade, placement of an implantable cardioverter-defibrillator (ICD), and preventive measures. Given his previous history of worsening arrhythmia with β-blockade and his desire to forgo ICD placement, he is currently managing his syndrome with preventive measures, which include daily potassium replacement and avoidance of all QTc-prolonging medications.

DISCUSSION

LQTS is a disorder of the cardiac myocardium that predisposes patients to sudden cardiac death. Torsades de pointes is a form of polymorphic ventricular tachycardia and is the cardiac arrhythmia most associated with LQTS. It is estimated to cause 3,000 to 4,000 sudden cardiac deaths in children annually [1]. LQTS can be classified as congenital or acquired, and the mechanism by which torsades de pointes develops in these 2 forms may differ, thus affecting the choice of pharmacologic therapy [2].

This complex physiologic process can be briefly summarized as follows:

- Congenital LQTS usually occurs after an adrenergic surge; therefore, it typically responds best to β-blockade, which is the mainstay of treatment [2,3].
- Acquired LQTS can occur in the context of delayed repolarization and bradycardia (usually drug induced), which prolong the repolarization phase with secondary lengthening of the QT interval. Along with removal of any offending drug therapies, the mainstay of treatment is IV magnesium and

therapies aimed at increasing the heart rate, which may include isoproter-enol, atropine, and glycopyrrolate (3,4).

- For both congenital and acquired LQTS, nonpharmacologic therapies that warrant consideration include cardiac pacing, which can be used for immediate short-term therapy and for long-term management. Pacing is particularly helpful for acquired LQTS after offending pharmacologic agents have been removed and magnesium and potassium levels have been corrected. Patients who have congenital LQTS but a previous adverse reaction to prior β-blockade therapy, such as the patient highlighted in the present case, can benefit from long-term pacing (5).

Patients with acquired LQTS may have an unknown congenital component, so further investigation into a possible congenital component to the LQTS should proceed after normal sinus rhythm has been restored (1). For patients with either congenital or acquired LQTS, the use of all QT-prolonging medications should be avoided and optimal electrolyte levels should be maintained at all times.

REFERENCES

1. Khan IA. Clinical and therapeutic aspects of congenital and acquired long QT syndrome. Am J Med. 2002 Jan;112(1):58–66.

2. Chiang CE. Congenital and acquired long QT syndrome: current concepts and management. Cardiol Rev. 2004 Jul-Aug;12(4):222–34.

3. Tan HL, Wilde AA, Peters RJ. Suppression of torsades de pointes by atropine. Heart. 1998 Jan;79(1):99–100.

4. Wehrens XH, Vos MA, Doevendans PA, Wellens HJ. Novel insights in the congenital long QT syndrome. Ann Intern Med. 2002 Dec 17;137(12):981–92.

5. Zipes DP, Camm AJ, Borggrefe M, Buxton AE, Chaitman B, Fromer M, et al; American College of Cardiology/American Heart Association Task Force; European Society of Cardiology Committee for Practice Guidelines; European Heart Rhythm Association; Heart Rhythm Society. ACC/AHA/ESC 2006 Guidelines for Management of Patients With Ventricular Arrhythmias and the Prevention of Sudden Cardiac Death: a report of the American College of Cardiology/American Heart Association Task Force and the European Society of Cardiology Committee for Practice Guidelines (writing committee to develop Guidelines for Management of Patients With Ventricular Arrhythmias and the Prevention of Sudden Cardiac Death): developed in collaboration with the European Heart Rhythm Association and the Heart Rhythm Society. Circulation. 2006 Sep 5;114(10):e385–484. Epub 2006 Aug 25.

The Kidneys Can See When the Eyes Cannot

SARAH J. LEE, MD, MPH, AND FLORANNE C. ERNSTE, MD

CASE PRESENTATION

A 16-year-old adolescent girl with no significant medical or family history presented with acute kidney failure, respiratory distress, and visual changes. Several weeks earlier, she had right-sided abdominal pain for 5 days. She did not have dysuria, hematuria, diarrhea, menorrhagia, nausea, or vomiting. At the local emergency department, abdominal ultrasonographic findings were reportedly normal. A pregnancy test was negative. She was given a diagnosis of constipation, and the pain resolved. Then she had malaise, fatigue, dry cough, sore throat, odynophagia, and painless blurry vision in her right eye with redness. Her primary care physician diagnosed a viral upper respiratory infection. However, the blurry vision progressed bilaterally by the following day. In the emergency department, she was diaphoretic, tachycardic (150 beats per minute), and hypertensive (blood pressure readings up to 200/130 mm Hg). Physical examination findings were unrevealing. Pertinent laboratory test findings are shown in Table 24.1.

The patient became bradycardic and hypoxic and required urgent intubation. The chest radiograph showed diffuse bilateral opacities. A dialysis catheter was placed, and the patient was transferred to a quaternary care medical center for further care. On arrival, a transthoracic echocardiogram showed the following: left

TABLE 24.1. Laboratory Test Results

Component	Finding
Hemoglobin, g/dL	9.0
Leukocyte count, ×10⁹/L	13.7
Neutrophils, %	87
Platelet count	Within reference range
Erythrocyte sedimentation rate, mm/h	114
Reticulocyte count, %	4.38
Haptoglobin, mg/dL	211
Serum anti–streptolysin O titer	Negative
Creatinine, mg/dL	5.0
Serum urea nitrogen, mg/dL	38
Electrolytes	
Bicarbonate, mmol/L	18
Other electrolytes	Within reference ranges
Lactate	Within reference range
Coagulation studies	
International normalized ratio	1.3
Activated partial thromboplastin time, s	26.7
Fibrinogen, mg/dL	550
Peripheral blood smear	No schistocytes
Urinalysis	
Bacteria	Negative
Erythrocytes	10-20
Casts	None

ventricular ejection fraction 30%, generalized left ventricular hypokinesis, a small amount of pericardial effusion, mild mitral valve regurgitation, moderate pulmonary valve regurgitation, and mild to moderate tricuspid valve regurgitation with an estimated right ventricular systolic pressure of 56 mm Hg.

Computed tomographic (CT) angiography showed occlusion of the abdominal aorta from the superior mesenteric artery origin to the aortic bifurcation, with an extensive collateral network in the anterior abdominal wall supplying the lower extremities, and occlusion of the renal arteries bilaterally with a right renal infarction. Consolidation was also seen in the lower lungs bilaterally.

Since the differential diagnosis included pulmonary-renal syndromes such as antineutrophil cytoplasmic autoantibody (ANCA)-associated vasculitides and

Goodpasture syndrome as well as systemic vasculitis, autoimmune serologies and a CT-guided percutaneous kidney biopsy were performed. The renal pathology findings were consistent with thrombotic microangiopathy with severe interstitial fibrosis and tubular atrophy. A diagnosis of primary catastrophic antiphospholipid syndrome (CAPS) associated with systemic lupus erythematosus (SLE) was made on the basis of the biopsy results; a positive antinuclear antibody titer of 1:120; positive double-stranded DNA (71.8 IU/mL); elevated levels of antibodies to β_2-glycoprotein 1 (immunoglobulin [Ig]G 21.9 units/mL, IgM 10.3 units/mL, and IgA 15.6 units/mL; reference ranges <10 units/mL); and elevated levels of antibodies to phospholipid (cardiolipin) antibodies (49.9 IgG phospholipid units, 37.2 IgM phospholipid units).

Therapeutic heparin anticoagulation was initiated for treatment of the thromboses related to CAPS and SLE. The patient received methylprednisolone 1 mg/kg for 3 days and a 7-day course of plasmapheresis followed by rituximab. Cyclophosphamide was not used because she had an acute kidney injury. She was slowly weaned from prednisone over several months, with the addition of mycophenolate mofetil, hydroxychloroquine, and trimethoprim-sulfamethizole prophylaxis.

She was extubated and switched to use of a nasal cannula soon after the first dose of corticosteroids and plasmapheresis. The blurry vision quickly resolved with control of the hypertension. A follow-up echocardiogram showed that the ejection fraction had improved from 30% to 49%. The residual mild reduction in systolic function was believed to be the result of autoimmune myocarditis.

Thrombolytics and surgery could precipitate showering of emboli to the single perfused kidney, so medical management with continuous heparin infusion was considered the safest option. This therapy was bridged to warfarin with a therapeutic goal international normalized ratio of 2.5 to 3.0 for lifelong anticoagulation. Six months after her initial presentation, the patient underwent aortobifemoral bypass grafting with thrombectomy of the right leg to create a target artery for attachment of a potential allograft. Surgery can trigger CAPS, so the patient was hospitalized for 4 days before the procedure to allow for bridging to heparin while warfarin was withheld. Because autoantibodies were present, anti–factor Xa levels were monitored instead of the activated partial thromboplastin time to ensure adequate anticoagulation. Heparin was titrated to achieve a goal anti–factor Xa level of 0.35 to 0.7 IU/mL. Anticoagulation was withheld the morning of surgery and resumed postoperatively. The patient had no complications as she transitioned back to therapeutic warfarin. Her outpatient oral immunosuppression regimen was continued perioperatively without a need for adjunctive immunosuppression.

The patient required hemodialysis for 11 months after her initial presentation. Then she received a deceased donor kidney transplant. She was able to return to high school 1 month after her transplant.

DISCUSSION

CAPS is an uncommon (<1% of patients), severe presentation in patients with antiphospholipid syndrome. Up to 50% of lupus patients have antiphospholipid antibodies. The most common triggers for CAPS are infection, neoplasia, oral contraceptives, trauma, surgery, and obstetric complications. CAPS is difficult to treat because of the rapid onset of vascular thrombosis in 3 or more systems, resulting in critical multiorgan failure (1).

Thrombotic microangiopathy is characterized by fibrin thrombi in glomeruli or arterioles (or both) and has been the most frequently reported intrarenal vascular lesion in antiphospholipid-positive patients with or without lupus, although overall it occurs infrequently (2). In patients with these lesions, antiphospholipid antibody testing is recommended. Other related conditions should be excluded (disseminated intravascular coagulation, thrombotic thrombocytopenic purpura–hemolytic uremic syndrome, HELLP syndrome, and ANCA-associated vasculitis) (3).

In patients with antiphospholipid syndrome and arterial thrombosis, an echocardiogram is recommended at the time of diagnosis (3). The prevalence of valvulopathy may be higher in patients with SLE and antiphospholipid syndrome (14%-86%), with mitral regurgitation as the most common abnormality. If the valves are abnormal, serial monitoring is recommended because surgery may be required in the future. One study found that patients with valvulopathy have a 93% likelihood of continued problems and may have worsening progression and that patients with normal valves have a 92% likelihood of remaining free of valvulopathy (4).

REFERENCES

1. Cervera R. Update on the diagnosis, treatment, and prognosis of the catastrophic antiphospholipid syndrome. Curr Rheumatol Rep. 2010 Feb;12(1):70–6.

2. Tektonidou MG, Sotsiou F, Nakopoulou L, Vlachoyiannopoulos PG, Moutsopoulos HM. Antiphospholipid syndrome nephropathy in patients with systemic lupus erythematosus and antiphospholipid antibodies: prevalence, clinical associations, and long-term outcome. Arthritis Rheum. 2004 Aug;50(8):2569–79.

3. Cervera R, Tektonidou MG, Espinosa G, Cabral AR, Gonzalez EB, Erkan D, et al. Task Force on Catastrophic Antiphospholipid Syndrome (APS) and non-criteria APS manifestations (I): catastrophic APS, APS nephropathy and heart valve lesions. Lupus. 2011 Feb;20(2):165–73.

4. Perez-Villa F, Font J, Azqueta M, Espinosa G, Pare C, Cervera R, et al. Severe valvular regurgitation and antiphospholipid antibodies in systemic lupus erythematosus: a prospective, long-term, followup study. Arthritis Rheum. 2005 Jun 15;53(3):460–7.

An Upper Airway Crisis

MAZEN O. AL-QADI, MBBS, AND MARK T. KEEGAN, MD

CASE PRESENTATION

A 54-year-old woman who had a past medical history of T-cell lymphoma was under evaluation for allogeneic bone marrow transplant when she presented with fever. Chest radiography showed a new pulmonary infiltrate. Bronchoscopy and bronchoalveolar lavage for microbiologic testing were planned. The patient had a documented lidocaine allergy; therefore, after administration of low-dose midazolam and ketamine, bronchoscopy was attempted without lidocaine topicalization. During an initial attempt to pass the bronchoscope through the vocal cords, inspiratory stridor developed with closure of the vocal cords and a concomitant decrease in oxygen saturation to 75%. A jaw thrust maneuver was performed, positive pressure ventilation (PPV) was applied with an anesthesia bag and mask, and additional sedative agents were administered. These interventions, coupled with placement of an endotracheal tube, restored the patency of the patient's airway. The patient's trachea was successfully extubated after the procedure without further complications.

DISCUSSION

Laryngospasm is a potentially life-threatening event that is characterized by spasm of the glottic muscles, which leads to reflex partial or complete upper airway obstruction. The glottic contraction is complex, and 3 types of laryngospasm are classically described (1,2):

1. *Expiratory stridor* is due to active adduction of the vocal cords. It rarely occurs with modern anesthetic techniques and drugs.
2. *Inspiratory stridor* is due to passive loss of abductor tone. The resultant pressure in the subglottic area is lower than atmospheric pressure, and the generated forceful airflow approximates the vocal cords during inspiration.
3. *Ball-valve obstruction* is due to laryngeal closure at the level of the true vocal cords, the false vocal cords, and the redundant supraglottic tissue. In contrast to the stridors (which are controlled by the intrinsic laryngeal muscles alone), ball-valve obstruction involves both intrinsic and extrinsic laryngeal muscles.

Contraction of the intrinsic laryngeal muscles is a protective reflex of the airway (during swallowing) that occurs through stimulation of the afferent fibers of the superior laryngeal nerve. Usually inhibited, it may be provoked by abnormal excitation, such as "light" anesthesia. Laryngospasm during anesthesia occurs in 8.7 per 1,000 anesthetic patients, with a higher incidence among children and infants (3). Clinically, laryngospasm manifests as an increase in the work of breathing with inspiratory or expiratory stridor and, when prolonged, hypoxemia and bradycardia, potentially leading to cardiac arrest. It may also give rise to negative-pressure pulmonary edema.

Risk factors for laryngospasm are classified as anesthesia-related, patient-related, and procedure-related (4). In the intensive care unit and the operating room, laryngospasm may be precipitated by manipulation of the airway (eg, laryngoscopy, suctioning, or extubation) or the application of a noxious stimulus (eg, intravenous line placement) when there is insufficient depth of anesthesia. Use of certain induction agents (eg, thiopental) and certain volatile anesthetic agents (eg, desflurane) are more likely to precipitate laryngospasm.

Laryngospasm is more common in patients with airway hyperactivity (due to asthma, smoking, or recent upper respiratory tract infection) and in patients with gastroesophageal reflux. It is more likely to occur in association with head or neck surgical procedures (eg, tonsillectomy or adenoidectomy).

Patients at greater risk of laryngospasm should be identified and preventive measures taken to minimize this serious complication (4). The most important consideration is the assurance of an adequate depth of anesthesia before airway

An Endocrine Emergency

W. BRIAN BEAM, MD,
AND OGNJEN GAJIC, MD

CASE PRESENTATION

A 61-year-old woman with a past medical history of type 2 diabetes mellitus and schizoaffective disorder presented with a 5-day history of abdominal pain, nausea, vomiting, loose stools, and decreased oral intake. Her husband said that she was using herbal remedies to treat her diabetes, although she had previously been prescribed insulin. She recently had contact with family members who had flulike symptoms.

Upon presentation to the emergency department, she was tachycardic, hypotensive, hypothermic (33.5°C), and minimally responsive. Blood samples were drawn for testing (Table 26.1). She was intubated for airway protection. She received volume resuscitation, potassium chloride, and intravenous antibiotics. Blood cultures were started. She was transferred to the intensive care unit (ICU). Upon examination in the ICU, she had been intubated, she was sedate, her mucosae were dry, her jugular veins were flat, the capillary refill was 3 seconds, and bowel sounds were normoactive. Her abdomen was soft with a palpable superficial midabdominal mass in association with a surgical scar. An abdominal radiograph showed moderately dilated loops of air-filled bowel in the central abdomen, which were concerning for a focal ileus. She was managed for diabetic ketoacidosis (DKA) according to a standardized protocol (3): Crystalloid resuscitation was continued with potassium replacement followed by an infusion of regular insulin.

TABLE 26.1. Summary of Patient's Laboratory Values at Presentation, Common Laboratory Values for DKA Patients on Admission, and Typical Electrolyte Deficits

Component	Patient at Presentation	Mean (SD) Values for Patients With DKA at Admission[1,2]	Typical Deficits at Presentation[1,2]
Glucose, mg/dL	395	616 (36)	. . .
Sodium, mmol/L	140	134 (1)	7-10 mEq/kg
Potassium, mmol/L	3.3	4.5 (0.13)	3-5 mEq/kg
Magnesium, mg/dL	1.6	. . .	1-2 mEq/kg
Phosphorus, mg/dL	2.7	. . .	5-7 mmol/kg
Calcium, ionized, mg/dL	5.3	. . .	1-2 mEq/kg
Serum urea nitrogen, mg/dL	21	32 (3)	. . .
Creatinine, mg/dL	0.5	1.1 (0.1)	. . .
pH	7.07	7.12 (0.04)	. . .
Bicarbonate, mmol/L	5	9.4 (1.4)	. . .
β-Hydroxybutyrate, mmol/L	7.1	9.1 (0.85)	. . .
Anion gap, mmol/L	22	17	. . .
Total osmolality, mOsm/kg	. . .	323 (2.5)	. . .
C-peptide, ng/mL	0.3	0.63 (0.09)	. . .
Human growth hormone, ng/mL	. . .	6.1 (1.2)	. . .
Cortisol, mcg/dL	. . .	18 (2)	. . .
Glucagon, pg/mL	. . .	580 (147)	. . .
Catecholamines, pg/mL	. . .	1.78 (0.4)	. . .
Leukocyte count, ×10^9/L	15.4	. . .	. . .
Hemoglobin A$_{1c}$, %	12.7	. . .	. . .
Water	. . .	. . .	6 L

Abbreviation: DKA, diabetic ketoacidosis.

Blood glucose, a basic metabolic panel, and arterial blood gas measurements were monitored every 2 hours. Eight hours after ICU admission, her blood glucose level was 204 mg/dL, and an infusion of dextrose 5% in water was initiated in addition to the insulin infusion. Despite adequate treatment of the DKA and normalization of the acidosis, she continued to require additional fluid resuscitation (a total of 14 L of fluid after admission) to maintain a mean arterial pressure greater than 60 mm Hg. When fluid replacement was considered adequate, low-dose norepinephrine infusion was started. A computed tomographic scan of the abdomen showed a small-bowel obstruction with a transition point. During exploratory laparotomy, a small-bowel torsion was found to be related to adhesions. The affected section of small bowel was resected, and an end-to-end anastomosis was performed. Postoperatively the patient was transferred back to the ICU, where the insulin infusion was continued, but the dextrose infusion was discontinued. She was later extubated and transitioned to a subcutaneous insulin regimen.

DISCUSSION

This patient's presentation is classic for DKA, which was likely triggered by a combination of her bowel obstruction and long-term nonadherence to her insulin regimen. DKA is the most common diabetes-related complication leading to ICU admission. This metabolic complication is triggered by a marked insulin deficiency along with elevated levels of counter-regulatory hormones. The result is an inability of insulin-sensitive tissues to use glucose, with accelerated gluconeogenesis and glycogenolysis followed by ketoacidosis. Hallmarks of the disorder include hyperglycemia, ketonemia, and an anion gap metabolic acidosis.

In diabetic patients, DKA is part of a spectrum of hyperglycemic emergencies, which also include hyperosmolar hyperglycemic state. Both emergencies are characterized by severe dehydration resulting from osmotic diuresis due to glucosuria, which leads to significant whole-body water and electrolyte deficits (Table 26.1). DKA is most common in patients with type 1 diabetes mellitus, but it can also occur in patients with type 2 diabetes mellitus. The most common precipitating factors are omission of insulin therapy and infection, but other causes should also be considered, such as myocardial infarction, medications (corticosteroids, thiazide diuretics, sympathomimetic agents, and second-generation cephalosporins), cocaine use, eating disorders, and mechanical problems with insulin pumps (4).

Physical examination findings consistent with dehydration are most common, but other common findings are Kussmaul respirations, acetone breath, emesis, and abdominal pain and tenderness. The abdominal pain usually has no visceral cause and the degree of pain usually correlates with the severity of the acidosis. Signs and symptoms mimic acute abdomen. Exploratory laparotomy is often negative in patients with DKA, but acute abdomen and DKA can occasionally coexist, as in the patient described above.

A preliminary diagnosis of DKA can be made if a patient has appropriate symptoms, hyperglycemia, and ketonuria. A basic metabolic panel, calcium, magnesium, phosphate, arterial blood gas values, β-hydroxybutyrate, hemoglobin A_{1c}, serum osmolality, and a complete blood cell count with a differential leukocyte count should also be obtained (Table 26.1 shows typical laboratory findings at admission). An electrocardiogram should be evaluated for rhythm abnormalities, and a urinalysis with urine culture and chest radiography should be considered to investigate for potential sources of infection. If a diabetic patient presents with a severely high anion gap metabolic acidosis without hyperglycemia, an alternative diagnosis should be considered (eg, ethylene glycol poisoning or bowel ischemia).

Management should focus on aggressive volume replacement with isotonic fluids, electrolyte repletion, and insulin replacement. Special attention should be given to potassium levels because a whole-body potassium deficit is common and hypokalemia may occur with insulin replacement. It is usually not necessary to treat mild hypophosphatemia. If phosphate is replaced, calcium levels should be monitored to avoid hypocalcemia. Bicarbonate replacement is usually not necessary unless the arterial pH is less than 6.9. Serial blood glucose, blood ketones, and basic metabolic panels should be monitored. Levels of β-hydroxybutyrate, the major ketone in DKA, should be measured where available. When the glucose level decreases to 200 to 250 mg/dL, an infusion of dextrose 5% in water should be added and insulin continued. This is necessary because glucose is required to metabolize ketone bodies. The dextrose can be discontinued when the patient's anion gap closes and serum ketone levels normalize. Patients can then be transitioned to a subcutaneous insulin regimen. Standardized protocols are useful for standardizing the management of complex fluid, glucose, insulin, and electrolyte situations and for preventing complications. In addition to treating DKA, a specific trigger should be sought both to assist in treatment and to help prevent future episodes (3). Consultation with a specialist in diabetes should be considered for further home-going recommendations and appropriate follow-up (5).

In summary, DKA is a common reason for ICU admission of diabetic patients. Patients present with hyperglycemia, ketonemia, and an anion gap metabolic acidosis. Prompt diagnosis, treatment, and a search for causation are the keys to successful management of these patients.

REFERENCES

1. Kitabchi AE, Nyenwe EA. Hyperglycemic crises in diabetes mellitus: diabetic ketoacidosis and hyperglycemic hyperosmolar state. Endocrinol Metab Clin North Am. 2006 Dec;35(4):725–51.

2. Kitabchi AE, Umpierrez GE, Miles JM, Fisher JN. Hyperglycemic crises in adult patients with diabetes. Diabetes Care. 2009 Jul;32(7):1335–43.

3. Bull SV, Douglas IS, Foster M, Albert RK. Mandatory protocol for treating adult patients with diabetic ketoacidosis decreases intensive care unit and hospital lengths of stay: results of a non-randomized trial. Crit Care Med. 2007 Jan;35(1):41–6.

4. Kitabchi AE, Umpierrez GE, Murphy MB, Barrett EJ, Kreisberg RA, Malone JI, et al. Management of hyperglycemic crises in patients with diabetes. Diabetes Care. 2001 Jan;24(1):131–53.

5. Nyenwe EA, Kitabchi AE. Evidence-based management of hyperglycemic emergencies in diabetes mellitus. Diabetes Res Clin Pract. 2011 Dec;94(3):340–51. Epub 2011 Oct 5.

Acute Renal Failure

MAZEN O. AL-QADI, MBBS, AND AMY W. WILLIAMS, MD

CASE PRESENTATION

An 84-year-old woman with a history of progressive chronic lymphocytic leukemia (with bulky lymph nodes) was admitted for chemotherapy with dexamethasone and rituximab. Several hours after receiving rituximab, she had severe respiratory distress. Physical examination was remarkable for new atrial fibrillation with rapid ventricular response (heart rate 130 beats per minute), respiratory rate 30 breaths per minute, blood pressure 100/55 mm Hg, 100% oxygen saturation at 2 L/min, bulky cervical lymphadenopathy, and splenomegaly. Laboratory test results included the following: leukocytes $3.4 \times 10^9/L$ (decreased from $28.5 \times 10^9/L$), sodium 130 mmol/L, potassium 6.5 mmol/L, calcium 8.2 mg/dL, phosphorous 7.2 mg/dL, bicarbonate 10 mmol/L, uric acid 12.2 mg/dL, and creatinine 1.9 mg/dL (increased from 1.0 mg/dL). Chest radiography showed bilateral infiltrates and a right pleural effusion.

Tumor lysis syndrome (TLS) was diagnosed on the basis of the Cairo-Bishop laboratory criteria (hyperkalemia, hyperphosphatemia, hyperuricemia, and hypocalcemia) and the Cairo-Bishop clinical criteria (renal impairment and arrhythmia) (Box 27.1) (1). The patient received 2 L of 0.9% normal saline, rasburicase, and broad-spectrum antibiotics for possible hospital-acquired pneumonia. Hemodialysis was deferred because of patient preference. The patient's condition

continued to deteriorate despite aggressive medical therapy, and she died after the family requested withdrawal of care.

DISCUSSION

TLS is a common emergency encountered in patients with hematologic malignancies. It is caused by the massive release of intracellular toxic metabolites when malignant tumor cells die (or by high rates of purine metabolism in spontaneous TLS). The syndrome develops within hours to days (up to 7 days) after initiation of chemotherapy and is characterized by hyperuricemia, hyperkalemia, hyperphosphatemia, and hypocalcemia. If not treated promptly, these metabolic derangements may result in acute kidney injury, metabolic acidosis, arrhythmias, and death.

The risk of TLS is greatest with large, rapidly growing, chemosensitive tumors such as B-cell acute lymphoblastic leukemia, acute myeloid leukemia (leukocyte count >75×10^9/L), and lymphoma with masses larger than 10 cm in diameter (particularly Burkitt lymphoma). Certain solid tumors (eg, hepatocellular carcinoma, prostate cancer, and small cell lung cancer) also carry the risk of TLS. Although TLS typically occurs after initiation of chemotherapy, it can occur spontaneously or after radiotherapy (2). Furthermore, TLS has been reported to occur in patients receiving corticosteroids for lymphoproliferative disorders, hormonal therapy for estrogen-receptor positive breast cancer, or biologic agents (eg, rituximab) for lymphoma and lymphoproliferative disorders (3,4).

Risk factors for the development of TLS in patients with hematologic malignancy include splenomegaly, elevated levels of lactate dehydrogenase, chronic kidney disease, and hyperuricemia before malignancy treatment. The massive release of intracellular contents results in a substantial imbalance of electrolytes with emergent hyperkalemia and hyperphosphatemia (Figure 27.1). Secondary hypocalcemia results from chelation of calcium with phosphorus. Subsequently, hyperkalemia and hypocalcemia can cause several serious complications, such as arrhythmias, seizures, and death. Kidney injury results from hyperuricemia due to metabolism of the liberated nucleic acids. Deposition of calcium-phosphate salts contributes to renal tubular and parenchymal injury as well. Acute kidney injury with a significant decrease in renal function further exacerbates the risk of significant ongoing hyperkalemia, hyperphosphatemia, hyperuricemia, and metabolic acidosis. The diagnosis of TLS is based on the Cairo-Bishop criteria (Box 27.1) (1).

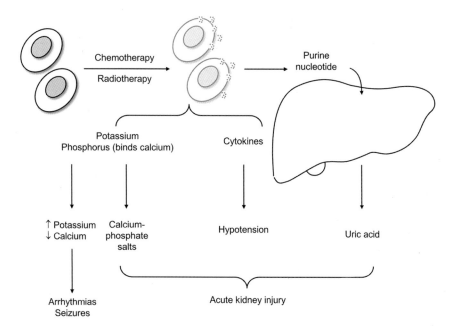

FIGURE 27.1. Pathophysiology of Tumor Lysis Syndrome. (Adapted from Tiu RV, Mountantonakis SE, Dunbar AJ, Schreiber MJ Jr. Tumor lysis syndrome. Semin Throbm Hemost. 2007 Jun;33[4]:397–407. Used with permission.)

BOX 27.1.
CAIRO-BISHOP CRITERIA FOR THE DIAGNOSIS OF TUMOR LYSIS SYNDROME (TLS)[a]

Laboratory criteria

1. Hyperuricemia (uric acid >8.0 mg/dL or ≥25% increase from baseline)
2. Hyperphosphatemia (phosphorus >4.5 mg/dL or ≥25% increase from baseline)
3. Hyperkalemia (potassium >6.0 mmol/L or ≥25% increase from baseline)
4. Hypocalcemia (calcium <7.0 mg/dL or ionized calcium <1.12 mg/dL)

Clinical criteria

1. Arrhythmias or sudden death due to hyperkalemia
2. Arrhythmias, sudden death, seizure, hypotension, or neuromuscular features (tetany, carpopedal spasm, Trousseau sign, Chvostek sign, or laryngospasm) due to hypocalcemia
3. Acute kidney injury (≥0.3 mg/dL increase in serum creatinine, creatinine >1.5 times baseline, or oliguria for ≥6 h)

---

[a] *The diagnosis of TLS requires at least 2 laboratory criteria during the same 24-hour period (≤3 days before or ≤7 days after initiation of chemotherapy or radiotherapy) and at least 1 clinical criterion.*

Adapted from Cairo and Bishop (1). Used with permission.

Treatment of TLS should focus on volume expansion to reestablish the normal concentrations of extracellular solutes. Intravenous fluids enhance urinary flow and, therefore, the excretion of potassium, phosphorus, and uric acid. In addition, aggressive hydration (with resulting urine output of 2.5-3.0 L daily) mitigates calcium-phosphate and urate crystal formation and tubular obstruction. Isotonic fluid (eg, normal saline) is recommended for replenishing intravascular volume in patients with TLS. Although it increases uric acid solubility, alkalinization of urine promotes xanthine crystallization and decreases calcium-phosphate solubility, so it is not recommended in the management of TLS (5).

Hypo-osmotic crystalloid (eg, 0.45% normal saline with 5% dextrose in water) can be used for maintenance of urine output. Furthermore, forced diuresis is needed if urine output remains inadequate (<150 mL/h) despite intravenous fluid therapy.

Xanthine oxidase inhibitors (eg, allopurinol or febuxostat) can be used to prevent hyperuricemia in patients at high risk of TLS by blocking the conversion of xanthine and hypoxanthine to uric acid. However, these agents are less effective after TLS has developed.

Rasburicase, a recombinant urate oxidase, is potent in metabolizing and converting uric acid to allantoin, which is very soluble and easily excreted in the urine. Rasburicase is the preferred agent in established TLS. Oxidative stress exerted by hydrogen peroxide (a metabolite of uric acid that is produced with the administration of rasburicase) may cause devastating hemolytic anemia and methemoglobinemia in patients who have glucose-6-phosphate dehydrogenase (G6PD) deficiency. Therefore, screening for G6PD deficiency is recommended before starting rasburicase.

Renal replacement therapy may be needed for patients who have metabolic abnormalities refractory to medical therapy, for patients who have acute kidney injury and anuria, or for patients who have heart failure and may not tolerate aggressive intravenous fluid administration. Moreover, early initiation of renal replacement therapy is recommended for life-threatening hyperkalemia (given the ongoing potassium release) and for severe hyperphosphatemia and hyperuricacidemia. Intermittent hemodialysis is the preferred renal replacement therapy because it is more effective than continuous methods in managing acute or emergent electrolyte abnormalities. Continuous renal replacement therapy may be needed after intermittent dialysis to prevent rebound hyperkalemia and hyperphosphatemia, especially in patients whose hemodynamic status is compromised.

REFERENCES

1. Cairo MS, Bishop M. Tumour lysis syndrome: new therapeutic strategies and classification. Br J Haematol. 2004 Oct;127(1):3–11.

2. Kaplan MA, Kucukoner M, Alpagat G, Isikdogan A. Tumor lysis syndrome during radiotherapy for prostate cancer with bone and bone marrow metastases without visceral metastasis. Ann Saudi Med. 2012 May-Jun;32(3):306–8.

3. Sparano J, Ramirez M, Wiernik PH. Increasing recognition of corticosteroid-induced tumor lysis syndrome in non-Hodgkin's lymphoma. Cancer. 1990 Mar 1;65(5):1072–3.

4. Francescone SA, Murphy B, Fallon JT, Hammond K, Pinney S. Tumor lysis syndrome occurring after the administration of rituximab for posttransplant lymphoproliferative disorder. Transplant Proc. 2009 Jun;41(5):1946–8.

5. Ten Harkel AD, Kist-Van Holthe JE, Van Weel M, Van der Vorst MM. Alkalinization and the tumor lysis syndrome. Med Pediatr Oncol. 1998 Jul;31(1):27–8.

Hypoxia and Diffuse Pulmonary Infiltrates in an Immunosuppressed Patient With Vasculitis

MATTHEW E. NOLAN, MD, AND ULRICH SPECKS, MD

CASE PRESENTATION

A 75-year-old woman has a history of antineutrophil cytoplasmic autoantibody (ANCA)–associated vasculitis (AAV) with cutaneous and renal involvement during immunosuppression, pulmonary blastomycosis, atrial fibrillation, deep vein thrombosis and pulmonary embolism during administration of warfarin, and breast cancer that is in remission. She was admitted to the intensive care unit because she had dyspnea, hypoxia, and diffuse pulmonary infiltrates.

Eighteen months before her current presentation she had a purpuric rash, hearing loss, arthralgias, and pauci-immune glomerulonephritis with elevated proteinase 3 (PR3)-ANCA titers, consistent with a diagnosis of AAV. She was treated with prednisone and cyclophosphamide followed by azathioprine, along with pneumocystis prophylaxis. She had no known pulmonary involvement with the vasculitis but was being treated for a pulmonary blastomycosis infection.

Two days before admission, the patient had a new episode of dyspnea without cough, hemoptysis, or fevers. She was admitted to the intensive care unit with hypoxia that was corrected with oxygen supplementation through a nonrebreather mask. Chest radiography showed bilateral diffuse perihilar alveolar infiltrates, and subsequent computed tomography showed diffuse upper lobe ground-glass opacities and lower lobe consolidation (Figure 28.1). An echocardiogram showed a left ventricular ejection fraction of 60% and a normal mitral valve. Laboratory test results are shown in Table 28.1. She was prescribed broad-spectrum antimicrobials, including antifungals.

The patient had refractory hypoxia with oxygen delivered at 15 L/min through a closed face mask (Pao_2 62 mm Hg), and she required intubation and mechanical ventilation shortly after arrival. Bronchoscopy did not show gross hemorrhage, but alveolar lavage produced a progressively blood-tinged return. Diagnostic evaluation included blood and alveolar fluid cultures and polymerase chain reaction (PCR) testing for bacteria, including acid-fast bacteria; viruses; and fungi, including *Pneumocystis*. Given the evidence supporting diffuse alveolar hemorrhage, and after the initial PCR studies were negative for viruses, the patient was treated with methylprednisolone 1,000 mg intravenously daily for 3 days (followed by prednisone 60 mg orally daily) and rituximab 375 mg/m² intravenously once weekly for 4 weeks as remission induction therapy for a severe

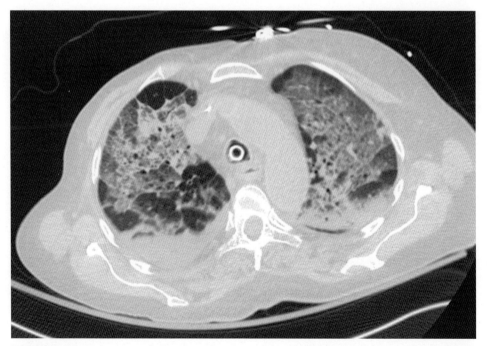

FIGURE 28.1. Computed Tomographic Scan After Intubation. The scan shows diffuse ground-glass opacities in the upper lung lobes with consolidation in the dependent lower lobes.

TABLE 28.1. Laboratory Test Results

Component	Result
Leukocyte count, ×10⁹/L	8.3
Neutrophils, %	92
Hemoglobin, g/dL	8.6
Platelet count	Within reference range
INR (during warfarin administration)	1.7
Erythrocyte sedimentation rate, mm/h	56
C-reactive protein, mg/L	132
ANCA	
Cytoplasmic ANCA	Positive
Proteinase 3 ANCA	Positive
Creatinine, mg/dL	
Baseline	1.2
Peak	1.9
Urinalysis (with microscopy)	Normal

Abbreviations: ANCA, antineutrophil cytoplasmic autoantibody; INR, international normalized ratio.

relapse of AAV. Her anticoagulation was reversed with fresh frozen plasma. She was extubated within 24 hours, and within 10 days she was breathing room air and showing improvement in her radiographic infiltrates. All the results from the infectious disease testing were negative.

DISCUSSION

Diffuse alveolar hemorrhage (DAH) is a clinical syndrome characterized by hypoxia and alveolar infiltrates due to blood filling the alveolar space from disruption of the alveolar-capillary interface. Anemia and hemoptysis are common but not necessary for the diagnosis; as in this case presentation, one-third of patients with DAH do not have hemoptysis at presentation (1). The organ-wide process of DAH must be distinguished from focal causes of pulmonary hemorrhage, such as tumors, bronchiectasis, or infections (2). Plain chest imaging shows an alveolar-type infiltrate, with computed tomography showing ground-glass opacification and possibly consolidation. The radiographic distribution of these abnormalities is often diffuse, but it can be focal or patchy (2,3).

Histopathologically, DAH is associated with pulmonary capillaritis, "bland" alveolar hemorrhage, or diffuse alveolar damage. However, because biopsy is not commonly performed, the associated clinical syndromes are most relevant. Pulmonary capillaritis is the most common cause and usually results from the ANCA-associated vasculitides (principally granulomatosis with polyangiitis [also called Wegener granulomatosis] and microscopic polyangiitis; rarely, eosinophilic granulomatosis with polyangiitis [also called Churg-Strauss syndrome]). Isolated pauci-immune pulmonary capillaritis, antiphospholipid syndrome, systemic lupus erythematosus, and other collagen-vascular diseases can also cause capillaritis. Bland alveolar hemorrhage is the predominant finding in anti–glomerular basement membrane antibody disease (also called anti-GBM nephritis or Goodpasture syndrome) and the only finding in mitral stenosis, coagulopathies, idiopathic pulmonary hemosiderosis, and rare drug-induced forms of DAH. Diffuse alveolar damage causing alveolar hemorrhage occurs in patients with acute respiratory disease syndrome, in bone marrow transplant recipients, and in persons who inhale toxins such as crack cocaine (1,3). The patient in this case presentation had a typical history for AAV and recently completed remission induction therapy. However, her PR3-ANCA positivity portends a higher risk of disease relapse compared to patients with myeloperoxidase ANCA (4).

DAH is a diagnosis of exclusion, and many predisposing conditions for DAH involve immunosuppressive therapy. Consequently, exclusion of infection is crucial when patients present with diffuse alveolar infiltrates. Bronchoscopy with alveolar lavage is usually necessary to rule out infection and rule in alveolar hemorrhage. The typical findings include a progressively bloody return with repeated lavage and the presence of hemosiderin-laden macrophages. Transbronchoscopic biopsies are often too small to confirm or exclude capillaritis, and video-assisted thoracoscopic lung biopsy is usually precluded because of the patient's tenuous respiratory status (3).

Laboratory testing for suspected DAH includes a complete blood cell count and an evaluation of coagulation markers to look for anemia or underlying coagulopathy. Kidney function tests and urinalysis may show concomitant renal involvement, a common feature especially in the vasculitides. Although in this case presentation, the patient had an acutely elevated creatinine value, the bland urine sediment was not consistent with active glomerulonephritis. Tests for inflammatory markers should be performed at baseline and then later to assess the treatment response. Autoantibody testing (ANCA, anti-GBM, and connective tissue serologies) should be performed in the appropriate clinical context to help establish a diagnosis (5).

Treatment of DAH first involves standard respiratory support, including mechanical ventilation, and reversing any underlying coagulopathy. The early initiation of high-dose glucocorticoids is the core of treatment in autoimmune-related DAH (ie, the vasculitides, connective tissue diseases, and anti-GBM nephritis), and this therapy may be started on the basis of clinical suspicion before infectious agent testing is complete. The typical therapy is methylprednisolone 1,000 mg daily for 3 to 5 days, followed by a slow tapering with prednisone over months. Adjuncts for immunosuppressive remission induction include cyclophosphamide, rituximab, or azathioprine. Plasmapheresis has a definite role in the treatment of anti-GBM nephritis and is under investigation for use in AAV. Recombinant factor VIIa has been used as salvage therapy for refractory alveolar hemorrhage (5).

DAH is a clinical syndrome characterized by hypoxia and alveolar infiltrates due to blood filling the alveolar space from disruption of the alveolar-capillary interface. Depending on the severity and acuity of the underlying disease, anemia and hemoptysis may be present or absent. The most common causes include an ANCA-associated vasculitis or connective tissue disease. Bronchoscopy should be performed to rule out infection and to rule in alveolar hemorrhage. Therapy with high-dose glucocorticoids and usually cyclophosphamide or rituximab should be started early if the cause of this life-threatening condition is an ANCA-associated vasculitis.

REFERENCES

1. Lara AR, Schwarz MI. Diffuse alveolar hemorrhage. Chest. 2010 May;137(5):1164–71.
2. Collard HR, Schwarz MI. Diffuse alveolar hemorrhage. Clin Chest Med. 2004 Sep;25(3):583–92.
3. Ioachimescu OC, Stoller JK. Diffuse alveolar hemorrhage: diagnosing it and finding the cause. Cleve Clin J Med. 2008 Apr;75(4):258, 260, 264–5 passim.
4. Specks U, Merkel PA, Seo P, Spiera R, Langford CA, Hoffman GS, et al; RAVE-ITN Research Group. Efficacy of remission-induction regimens for ANCA–associated vasculitis. N Engl J Med. 2013 Aug 1;369(5):417–27.
5. Krause ML, Cartin-Ceba R, Specks U, Peikert T. Update on diffuse alveolar hemorrhage and pulmonary vasculitis. Immunol Allergy Clin North Am. 2012 Nov;32(4):587–600. Epub 2012 Sep 28.

A Paraneoplastic Syndrome

ANDRES BORJA ALVAREZ, MD,
AND EMIR FESTIC, MD

CASE PRESENTATION

A 69-year-old Vietnamese woman with a previous diagnosis of grade 1 follicular lymphoma was admitted with a 4-month history of shortness of breath with wheezing and a nocturnal cough treated initially with inhaled fluticasone-salmeterol. Oral thrush developed and progressed to mucositis, which was treated with topical nystatin and lidocaine. She was taking no other pertinent medications. She also complained of gradually worsening weakness of her arms and legs, difficulty with standing and walking, decreased appetite, and an 11.4-kg weight loss. She said that she did not have fever, chills, nausea, vomiting, constipation, diarrhea, joint pain, swelling, or rash. She was admitted to another hospital for pneumonia, hypercapnic respiratory failure, and gram-positive sepsis. When she could not be weaned from the ventilator, she was transferred to a tertiary care facility, where broad-spectrum antibiotics were continued and, despite bronchoscopy showing significant mucopurulent secretions, bronchoalveolar lavage culture results were negative.

On physical examination, the patient was intubated and minimally sedated; she had a slight decrease of breath sounds in the right lower lobe without crackles or wheezing. Strength was preserved in all extremities, cranial nerve function was normal, and deep tendon reflexes were increased with clonus more prominent in the lower extremities. The other physical examination findings were normal. Initial attempts to wean her from the ventilator were unsuccessful.

Laboratory data showed compensated hypercapnia with adequate compensation, mild anemia and thrombocytosis, normal electrolyte levels, low creatine kinase levels, and high levels of λ and κ free light chains. Chest radiography showed the endotracheal tube in an appropriate location and clear lung fields without consolidation. Computed tomographic angiography was negative for pulmonary embolism and showed no evidence of parenchymal lung disease. Results of electromyography with a nerve conduction study were normal, and magnetic resonance imaging showed only an incidental capillary telangiectasia in the pons and mild generalized cerebral atrophy. A paraneoplastic screen showed an anti-acetylcholine muscle-binding antibody.

The patient tolerated a T-piece trial and was extubated, but then she became lethargic with respiratory distress. Blood gas measurements showed hypercapnia despite bilevel positive airway pressure support. The patient was reintubated, but she could not be weaned from mechanical support because she had high pressure support requirements and low negative inspiratory force.

DISCUSSION

Paraneoplastic neurologic syndromes (PNSs) are rare effects of cancer that are not caused by a tumor or its metastasis, an infection, or a metabolic process (1). PNS requires a high level of awareness because it can be the initial manifestation of a malignant process, and it can affect the nervous system at any level.

The pathogenesis of PNS is related to an autoimmune response. The discovery of multiple antibodies led to the understanding that antigens in the nervous system can be abnormally expressed by a tumor. The role of each antibody has not been completely characterized, and the absence of antibodies does not rule out the diagnosis of PNS. In some cases, the antibodies might be only a marker of the immune process and not the actual cause.

Certain classic PNSs should be remembered. The most common is Lambert-Eaton syndrome, a presynaptic disorder with weakness that improves after repetitive stimulation. Another example is subacute cerebellar ataxia, which is characterized by ataxia, a wide-base gait, and often nystagmus (2). A syndrome that occurs almost exclusively in patients with small cell lung cancer is characterized by decreased visual acuity and photosensitivity. In other syndromes, such as dermatomyositis, myasthenia gravis, encephalomyelitis, and sensory neuropathy, the symptoms reflect the affected area.

Although the presentation of these diseases is not specific for PNS and the syndromes described above are not the exclusive presentation of PNSs, these diseases and syndromes should prompt a search for malignancy. Dermatomyositis is a good example because the various presentations and the timing of PNS make the diagnosis particularly difficult (sometimes months to years pass before the malignancy is apparent). A high level of awareness will help with the clinical diagnosis that may lead to the appropriate treatment.

Any malignancy can present with PNSs, and small cell lung cancer and lymphoma (especially Hodgkin type) are frequent causes of PNSs. Other associated malignancies are breast cancer, gynecologic cancer, and melanoma. The appropriate workup includes computed tomography of the chest, abdomen, and pelvis and mammography. The paraneoplastic antibody screen and tumor markers should be included if no obvious cause is found. The search for malignancy depends on the individual patient and the patient's nonmodifiable and modifiable risk factors.

If PNS is suspected, the presence of a series of antibodies can aid in the diagnosis. One antibody, for example, is Hu-Ab, which is related to small cell lung carcinoma and PNS. Other PNS-related antibodies include Yo-Ab, CV2-Ab, Ri-Ab, amphiphysin-Ab, Tr-Ab, Ma2-Ab, and CAR-Ab; however, negative antibody results do not exclude the diagnosis, and a high level of awareness must guide the diagnosis.

In some patients, the symptoms of PNS are relieved or improved by treating the underlying malignancy. Medications for patients with myasthenia gravis include pyridostigmine, corticosteroids, and steroid-sparing agents (eg, azathioprine). The treatment may include the use of plasmapheresis or intravenous immunoglobulins for acute PNS or exacerbations (3). The treatment of lymphoma in some cases may lead to improvement of PNS symptoms.

For the patient in this case presentation, the diagnosis of follicular lymphoma preceded the presentation of paraneoplastic-like syndrome. The absence of another specific cause for the hypercapnic respiratory failure pointed toward PNS. While identification of potential specific antibodies was pending, supportive treatment with mechanical ventilation with a tracheostomy continued.

There are no data specific to intensive care unit monitoring of patients with impending respiratory failure from PNS. However, practical and useful information can be extrapolated from patients with neuromuscular disease. In a 2009 Mayo Clinic review of patients with Guillain-Barré syndrome, the authors identified early markers of impending respiratory failure (3). These include vital capacity less than 20 mL/kg, negative inspiratory force or maximal inspiratory pressure less than 40 cm H_2O, and a 30% decrease in baseline vital capacity. Therefore, these patients should be monitored in the intensive care unit with frequent reassessments.

The ideal mode of mechanical ventilation should be based on the experience of the prescribing physician. For long-term therapy, evidence indicates that non-invasive positive pressure ventilation (NIPPV) prolongs life and increases quality of life of patients who have neuromuscular diseases, broadly including PNS in the etiology. For short-term care, there is no evidence that supports or rejects its use. Therapy should be individualized for each patient because NIPPV can improve oxygenation and hypercarbia, but it may increase the risk of aspiration. A trial of NIPPV should be relatively short, so that improvement is reassessed in a matter of hours. If there is no improvement, the patient should be intubated and mechanical ventilation instituted to prevent worse outcomes associated with delayed mechanical ventilation.

Many authors have tried to identify the ideal time for tracheostomy, but it remains unclear. Neurologic disease–related respiratory failure is a risk factor for tracheostomy (4). The time of tracheostomy has not been shown to alter the duration of ventilation or the mortality rate. In patients with neuromuscular disease, tracheostomy allows for better quality of life by permitting decreased sedation and increased activity and speech.

PNSs are associated with multiple malignancies that often precede them (most frequently, lymphoid malignancies and small cell lung cancer). A high level of clinical awareness is crucial for the clinical diagnosis of PNS, and patients should be closely monitored for bulbar dysfunction, negative inspiratory force, and vital capacity. Tracheostomy should be considered for patients who will require prolonged ventilatory support, for patients who undergo multiple intubations, and for patients who have neurologic disease that prompts mechanical ventilation.

REFERENCES

1. Honnorat J, Antoine JC. Paraneoplastic neurological syndromes. Orphanet J Rare Dis. 2007 May 4;2:22.

2. Shimazu Y, Minakawa EN, Nishikori M, Ihara M, Hashi Y, Matsuyama H, et al. A case of follicular lymphoma associated with paraneoplastic cerebellar degeneration. Intern Med. 2012;51(11):1387–92. Epub 2012 Jun 1.

3. Lawn ND, Fletcher DD, Henderson RD, Wolter TD, Wijdicks EF. Anticipating mechanical ventilation in Guillain-Barré syndrome. Arch Neurol. 2001 Jun;58(6):893–8.

4. Frutos-Vivar F, Esteban A, Apezteguia C, Anzueto A, Nightingale P, Gonzalez M, et al; International Mechanical Ventilation Study Group. Outcome of mechanically ventilated patients who require a tracheostomy. Crit Care Med. 2005 Feb;33(2):290–8.

Complicated Diarrheal Illness

ARJUN GUPTA, MBBS, AND SAHIL KHANNA, MBBS

CASE PRESENTATION

An 80-year-old man with a history of glaucoma, inguinal hernia, and benign prostatic hypertrophy was admitted with a 4-day history of abdominal pain and diarrhea (7 watery, nonbloody bowel movements daily). Two weeks before admission, he received amoxicillin-clavulanic acid for 10 days for a skin infection. He was tachycardic and afebrile, and he had abdominal tenderness. Laboratory test results for leukocyte count, electrolytes, creatinine, and albumin were unremarkable. Polymerase chain reaction (PCR) analysis of stool was positive for *Clostridium difficile*, and intravenous metronidazole 500 mg 3 times daily was initiated. The diarrhea improved, and the frequency decreased to 3 times daily in 3 days. The patient was discharged with a 14-day course of oral metronidazole. Two weeks after he completed the course of metronidazole, he presented with increasing abdominal cramps and diarrhea (6-7 watery stools daily); a 14-day course of oral vancomycin was prescribed with symptom resolution.

Subsequently, 4 weeks after finishing the vancomycin, the patient presented with severe diarrhea; abdominal pain; dizziness; nonbilious, nonbloody emesis; and a 9.1-kilogram weight loss. He was febrile and hypotensive, and he had severe abdominal tenderness. His leukocyte count was 30.6×10^9/L. Computed tomography of the abdomen, which was performed to rule out a perforation or abscess, showed severe pancolitis. He was admitted to the medical intensive care unit for severe sepsis and treated with aggressive hydration, intravenous metronidazole 500 mg every 8 hours, and oral vancomycin 500 mg every 6 hours. PCR analysis of stool for *C difficile* was positive, and a workup for infectious agents was otherwise negative. The patient remained hypotensive despite phenylephrine administration, and he received several liters of crystalloid infusion, which led to a hyperchloremic metabolic acidosis; the serum lactate level was normal. His condition stabilized within 24 hours, and he was transferred to the general medical unit. The leukocyte count improved to 12.2×10^9/L, and the plan included a 14-day course of oral vancomycin and intravenous metronidazole, followed by vancomycin tapered over 7 weeks. However, he continued to have diarrhea and abdominal pain, and the leukocyte count increased to 18.2×10^9/L on hospital day 5.

Vancomycin failure was suspected, and the patient declined colectomy, so fecal microbiota transplantation (FMT) was performed. Because the patient had ileus, a complete bowel preparation was deferred. After 2 enemas with tap water, 50 g of donor stool was diluted and filtered in 250 mL normal saline and infused into the transverse colon with a flexible sigmoidoscope. The colon had severe diffuse inflammation with pseudomembranes. Symptoms improved, with reduced abdominal pain and stool frequency, and the leukocyte count normalized. Three days after FMT, PCR analysis of stool for *C difficile* was negative. The patient was discharged to a nursing home without antibiotics.

The patient presented 1 week later with severe diarrhea, dehydration, abdominal pain, and leukocytosis (22.7×10^9/L). Abdominal radiography suggested ileus but no free intra-abdominal air. PCR analysis of stool was positive for *C difficile* toxin. He was readmitted with a diagnosis of severe-complicated *C difficile* infection (CDI), and therapy was reinitiated with intravenous metronidazole and oral vancomycin. However, he did not improve clinically, and the leukocytosis worsened (38.9×10^9/L). He declined surgical intervention or another FMT, so he was discharged home with hospice care, where he died 1 week later.

DISCUSSION

CDI is the most common cause of infectious diarrhea in hospitalized patients (1) and has surpassed methicillin-resistant *Staphylococcus aureus* as the most common cause of nosocomial infection. CDI is being identified increasingly in community patients without prior hospitalization or antibiotic exposure. Traditional risk factors include older age, antibiotic exposure, and hospitalization; newer risk factors are being identified, although the role of gastric acid suppression is still controversial (2). Treatment recommendations for CDI are based on severity, and patients with severe or severe-complicated CDI should receive aggressive therapy to prevent adverse outcomes.

When patients have CDI, it is important to distinguish between severe CDI and severe-complicated CDI to promptly initiate intensive or surgical therapy. Complications of CDI include shock, toxic megacolon, perforation, colectomy, and death. The Infectious Diseases Society of America guidelines classify CDI as *severe* if the leukocyte count is more than $15 \times 10^9/L$ or if the serum creatinine level increases by 50% or more from baseline and as *severe-complicated* if CDI is associated with hypotension, sepsis, ileus, toxic megacolon perforation, a need for admission to the intensive care unit, a need for surgical intervention, or death (3).

Metronidazole 500 mg orally 3 times daily for 10 to 14 days is used for mild-moderate CDI, and oral vancomycin 125 mg 4 times daily for 10 to 14 days is used for severe CDI. Patients with severe-complicated CDI are treated with intravenous metronidazole 500 mg every 8 hours, oral vancomycin (500 mg 4 times daily), and possibly rectal vancomycin (3). Surgical intervention is indicated for severe-complicated CDI that does not respond to antibiotic therapy or if the patient has toxic megacolon, colonic perforation, or acute abdomen. Colectomy is associated with high perioperative mortality and the need for a permanent ileostomy. In a small retrospective study (4) of an alternative surgical technique involving intra-operative colonic lavage and postoperative vancomycin enemas after creation of a diverting ileostomy, mortality was markedly reduced (compared to mortality with colectomy), with more than 90% of patients also retaining their colon. Early surgical intervention can be lifesaving for severely ill patients with septic shock due to CDI. FMT, which has a success rate of 90%, is reserved for patients with recurrent CDI and sometimes for those with severe CDI that does not respond to conventional medical therapy (5).

The patient in this case presentation was initially treated appropriately with oral metronidazole when he presented with mild-moderate CDI. Recurrent CDI occurs in up to 20% to 40% of patients and is more common in the elderly and in those receiving concomitant systemic antibiotics. The patient was adequately treated with a combination of metronidazole and vancomycin for severe-complicated CDI, but the treatment failed after an initial response to antibiotics and FMT. FMT failure was likely due to suboptimal bowel preparation and stool administration and the presence of severe-complicated CDI. Although FMT has a very high success rate (>90%), procedural differences in bowel preparation, route of administration, donor selection, stool processing, underlying CDI severity, and number of instillations may influence outcomes. As in this patient, severe-complicated CDI is associated with high morbidity and mortality despite aggressive management, especially in the elderly (1,3). Early surgical intervention should be considered for all patients with severe-complicated CDI.

REFERENCES

1. Khanna S, Pardi DS. *Clostridium difficile* infection: new insights into management. Mayo Clin Proc. 2012 Nov;87(11):1106–17.

2. Khanna S, Pardi DS. Gastric acid suppression and *Clostridium difficile* infection: is there a causal connection? Clin Gastroenterol Hepatol. 2012 May;10(5):564. Epub 2012 Jan 2.

3. Cohen SH, Gerding DN, Johnson S, Kelly CP, Loo VG, McDonald LC, et al; Society for Healthcare Epidemiology of America; Infectious Diseases Society of America. Clinical practice guidelines for *Clostridium difficile* infection in adults: 2010 update by the society for healthcare epidemiology of America (SHEA) and the infectious diseases society of America (IDSA). Infect Control Hosp Epidemiol. 2010 May;31(5):431–55.

4. Neal MD, Alverdy JC, Hall DE, Simmons RL, Zuckerbraun BS. Diverting loop ileostomy and colonic lavage: an alternative to total abdominal colectomy for the treatment of severe, complicated *Clostridium difficile* associated disease. Ann Surg. 2011 Sep;254(3):423–7.

5. Gough E, Shaikh H, Manges AR. Systematic review of intestinal microbiota transplantation (fecal bacteriotherapy) for recurrent *Clostridium difficile* infection. Clin Infect Dis. 2011 Nov;53(10):994–1002.

Persistent Shock With Hemorrhagic Complications

SANGITA TRIVEDI, MBBS,
RAHUL KASHYAP, MBBS,
AND MICHAEL E. NEMERGUT, MD, PHD

CASE PRESENTATION

A 6-year-old, 24-kg boy without a significant past medical history presented to the emergency department with a 4-day history of fever, myalgias, and generalized rash with prominent facial flushing. On the day of admission, his symptoms were notable for the appearance of diffuse petechiae and periods of profound irritability with abdominal pain and vomiting. He recently returned from a family vacation in Puerto Rico.

On presentation, he had normothermia, mild tachycardia, tachypnea, and normal blood pressure, albeit a narrow pulse pressure. His extremities were cool and poorly perfused, with a capillary refill time of 4 seconds. His mentation was normal, and mild epigastric tenderness was elicited on examination. The blood cell count was significant for leukopenia, thrombocytopenia (platelets, $30 \times 10^9/$ L), and a relatively high hematocrit. The coagulation profile showed a normal pro-thrombin time, mild hypofibrinoginemia, and mild prolongation of the activated partial thromboplastin time. Chest radiography showed bilateral, lower lobe infil-trates and a small right-sided pleural effusion. The differential diagnosis included septic shock, viral hemorrhagic fever, and leukemia. Appropriate culture and serologic studies were started, fluids were given in boluses, and broad-spectrum antibiotics were administered. Abdominal ultrasonography, for evaluating the epigastric tenderness, showed gallbladder wall edema and ascites.

Within hours after the patient was admitted, profound hypotension, respiratory failure, and encephalopathy rapidly developed. Additional crystalloid boluses were administered without resolution of the shock, and the child was subsequently intubated for respiratory failure with associated metabolic acidosis, hyperlactatemia, and fluid-refractive shock. Chest radiography showed a significant increase in the size of the pleural effusion.

Invasive hemodynamic monitoring showed a low central venous pressure, arterial hypotension with overt variability with the respiratory cycle, and oliguria. Despite prior aggressive volume resuscitation, the blood cell count continued to suggest hemoconcentration with a high hematocrit. Laboratory evaluation showed worsening thrombocytopenia (platelets, 10×10^9/L), hypoalbuminemia, and elevated hepatic transaminases. The persistent hypotension and capillary leakage prompted additional fluid resuscitation with 5% albumin. Serologic evaluation showed a positive result for dengue virus.

Blood pressure and central venous pressure improved in response to continued resuscitation, and the hematocrit level stabilized. The albumin infusion rate of 10 mL/kg/h was continued for 2 hours, and then the fluids were switched to normal saline at 5 mL/kg/h. The hematocrit was checked before and after fluid boluses and also every 2 hours for management of fluid therapy.

After a few hours of apparent hemodynamic stability, prominent bleeding was observed from the gastric tube, rectum, trachea, and cannulation site. The hematocrit decreased to the low end of the reference range, and the platelet count decreased to 5×10^9/L, the hepatic enzyme values increased, and the coagulation profile suggested disseminated intravascular coagulation. Because of his ongoing blood loss, the patient was given a transfusion of packed red blood cells, platelets, and vitamin K. His hematocrit did not respond to the initial transfusion, so another packed red blood cell transfusion was given and was followed by a normal saline infusion, as recommended by the World Health Organization (WHO) protocol for treatment of dengue shock syndrome (also called dengue hemorrhagic fever) (1).

Over the next 24 hours, the patient's hemodynamic and perfusion status normalized; however, he had a further increase in infiltrates and pleural effusion on chest radiography. The patient's weight increased by 2.5 kg compared to his weight at admission, and the increase was thought to be related to the aggressive volume resuscitation. He was subsequently given diuretics and, after his cardiorespiratory status improved, he was extubated the next day.

DISCUSSION

The dengue virus is transmitted to humans by mosquitoes in the genus *Aedes*. Patients with dengue viral infection present with a spectrum of illness ranging from asymptomatic to fatal. The severe form, dengue shock syndrome, is primarily a disease of infants and children and is characterized by shock, multiorgan system dysfunction, and bleeding (1). The disease is endemic in Puerto Rico, where the most recent islandwide epidemic occurred in 2007, when more than 10,000 cases were diagnosed (2). WHO estimates that 50,000 cases of dengue shock syndrome occur annually and 22,000 deaths occur annually among children worldwide (3). The pathogenesis of the disease is not completely clear; however, in severe disease, markedly increased vascular permeability leads to shock. The clinical manifestation of the disease occurs in 3 phases.

Phase 1, the *febrile phase*, is characterized by high-grade fever and nonspecific symptoms that include headache, nausea, vomiting, myalgias, arthralgias, and generalized rash for 2 to 7 days.

Phase 2, the *critical phase*, starts with defervescence and is characterized by leukopenia, thrombocytopenia, and plasma leakage, with a corresponding increase in the hematocrit; these features are used to monitor the severity of the disease. Phase 2 lasts for 24 to 48 hours, and the extent of plasma loss dictates the clinical severity of the disease. Typically, the hypovolemic shock observed in this phase is compensated. The systolic blood pressure may be normal, and the diastolic blood pressure may even be elevated until late; the patient often remains alert until sudden decompensation. Prolonged shock, acidosis, and thrombocytopenia set the stage for disseminated intravascular coagulation, with bleeding typically from the gastrointestinal tract. The difficulties in management arise mainly in this stage from the marked hemodynamic instability that is associated with large volume shifts and hemorrhage. Fluid therapy must be tailored to keep pace with the evolution of the clinical course. The guidelines for management are different from those for managing septic shock (4). Associated with unstable vital signs, an increasing hematocrit indicates the need to administer fluids, but a low hematocrit suggests occult hemorrhage or the need for transfusion (if <30%). The therapeutic end points are normalization of a low systolic blood pressure, a pulse pressure of more than 30 mm Hg, urine output of more than 0.5 to 1 mL/kg/h, and a gradual decrease in high hematocrit levels (1,5).

Phase 3, the *recovery phase,* lasts for 2 to 3 days and is marked by absorption of the leaked plasma into intravascular space, stable blood pressure, and diuresis. Hematologic values start reverting to the reference range. A low hematocrit, stable vital signs, and urine output of more than 1.5 to 2 mL/kg/h may be the earliest indicators for weaning the patient from fluid replacement and preventing overload that might cause pulmonary edema and tense large-volume ascites. Prophylactic blood products should not be used in patients who are not bleeding (1,5).

Appropriate hydration as the disease progresses is the mainstay of acute management and resuscitation. The 2-pronged strategy includes early recognition and intervention for shock management and judicious fluid management to prevent fluid overload.

REFERENCES

1. Handbook for clinical management of dengue [Internet]. Geneva: World Health Organization; c2012. [cited 2015 Sep 11]. Available from: http://apps.who.int/iris/bitstream/10665/76887/1/9789241504713_eng.pdf?ua=1.

2. Dengue [Homepage on the Internet]. Atlanta (GA): Centers for Disease Control and Prevention. [updated 2014 Jun 9; cited 2015 Sep 11]. Available from: http://www.cdc.gov/dengue/epidemiology/index.html.

3. Impact of dengue [Internet]. Geneva: World Health Organization; c2015. [cited 2015 Sep 11]. Available from: http://www.who.int/crs/disease/dengue/impact/en/.

4. Dellinger RP, Levy MM, Rhodes A, Annane D, Gerlach H, Opal SM, et al; Surviving Sepsis Campaign Guidelines Committee including the Pediatric Subgroup. Surviving Sepsis Campaign: international guidelines for management of severe sepsis and septic shock: 2012. Crit Care Med. 2013 Feb;41(2):580–637.

5. Ranjit S, Kissoon N. Dengue hemorrhagic fever and shock syndromes. Pediatr Crit Care Med. 2011 Jan;12(1):90–100.

An Unusual Presentation of Disseminated Histoplasmosis

LOKENDRA THAKUR, MBBS, AND VIVEK IYER, MD, MPH

CASE PRESENTATION

A 41-year-old man presented to the internal medicine outpatient clinic for evaluation of fever of 6 weeks' duration. While there, he was uncomfortable and appeared ill; he was febrile and hypotensive. He was sent to the emergency department and, after initial workup and stabilization, he was admitted to the medical intensive care unit (ICU) for further management. Additional history included generalized weakness and fatigue with multiple admissions and treatment with intravenous antibiotics and fluids in the preceding 6 weeks. He responded each time to antibiotic therapy, although microbiologic cultures were negative. An echocardiogram and other imaging studies performed elsewhere did not help to identify a source of infection. He had a skin ulcer on the left elbow and a leg wound that appeared to be superficial and had yielded methicillin-sensitive *Staphylococcus aureus* in a previous culture. He was morbidly obese and gave a history of long-term, low-dose corticosteroid use for the past 20 years to treat asthma. He also gave a history of recurrent joint pain localized to the small joints, which was evaluated at another facility and was described as nonrheumatic.

On examination he was hypotensive (blood pressure 84/47 mm Hg) and slightly tachycardic (heart rate 102 beats per minute), and he had a normal respiratory rate and oxygen saturation while breathing room air. He appeared anxious and fatigued with dry mucous membranes, a cushingoid appearance with central obesity, striae, neck fat pad, and rounded facies. Other significant findings on examination included the presence of a soft tissue infection in his left leg, buttock, and left elbow area, with mild edema in the lower extremities. He had tenderness over the left gluteal region and dystrophic toenails. His mentation was normal, and his cranial nerves were intact. His muscle strength was equal bilaterally, and findings on systemic examination of his heart, lung, and abdomen were unremarkable.

Results of a chemistry panel included hyponatremia (133 mmol/L) and an elevated creatinine (1.7 mg/dL). Initial imaging studies included a computed tomogram of the abdomen and pelvis, which showed evidence of left gluteal cellulitis and abscess.

The patient was treated with vancomycin, cefepime, metronidazole, and aggressive fluid resuscitation. His hemodynamic status improved, and infectious disease and rheumatology specialists were consulted in the first 2 days of the ICU stay. Further investigations were pending when he was transferred to a general medicine unit for further investigations and management. The patient's fever recurred during de-escalation of antibiotics, and the coverage was broadened, but his constitutional status and hemodynamic status remained poor, so he was transferred back to the ICU. Further interventions were ordered to find the source of infection and to look for an atypical cause of the persistent high-grade fever. A hematologist was consulted when the patient became leukopenic and thrombocytopenic. White blood cell scanning with indium In 111 showed a multifocal soft tissue infection in the medial left upper thigh. Viral testing, including testing for human immunodeficiency virus, was negative.

The patient's elevated ferritin level (37,630 mcg/L) prompted the performance of a bone marrow biopsy, which showed hemophagocytosis. The patient was transferred to the inpatient hematology-oncology unit, where chemotherapy was initiated with cyclosporine, etoposide, and corticosteroids. While he was undergoing chemotherapy, results from a subcutaneous fluid culture from the left thigh were reported as positive for *Histoplasma capsulatum*. Chemotherapy was stopped and his medication was switched to intravenous amphotericin B for histoplasmosis. Renal failure developed, so amphotericin B was switched to itraconazole. While he was receiving itraconazole, he showed signs of liver failure and underwent liver biopsy. Liver biopsy showed features of hemophagocytosis and narrow-based budding yeasts within the sinusoids, which were consistent with *Histoplasma* species. He was switched back to amphotericin B infusion with a plan to start lifelong oral itraconazole after his liver enzymes normalized. He gradually improved, although he remained weak and required a percutaneous endoscopic gastrostomy tube for nutrition.

DISCUSSION

Hemophagocytic lymphohistiocytosis (HLH) is divided into primary (genetic) and secondary (acquired) forms. The familial form is an autosomal recessive disorder with an incidence of 1 in 50,000 live births. It is occasionally associated with mutations in the perforin gene, it often occurs during early childhood, and without treatment it is usually fatal within 2 months after the onset of symptoms (1). Clinical presentation is similar to that for severe sepsis and septic shock. In this patient, the profoundly elevated serum ferritin level (37,630 mcg/L) led to the suspicion of HLH. The triglyceride levels were normal, but the bone marrow biopsy showed hemophagocytosis (2).

In 1994, the Histiocyte Society initiated a prospective international collaborative therapeutic study (HLH-94), which stated that the diagnosis of HLH is based on 5 criteria (fever, splenomegaly, cytopenia affecting ≥2 lineages in the peripheral blood, hypertriglyceridemia or hypofibrinoginemia or both, and hemophagocytosis). The Histiocyte Society added 3 more criteria in 2004 (HLH-2004): 1) low or absent natural killer cell activity, 2) hyperferritinemia, and 3) high levels of soluble interleukin (IL)-2–receptor (3). Five of the 8 criteria must be fulfilled to diagnose HLH. This patient had fever, leukopenia, hemophagocytosis, hyperferritinemia, and mild splenomegaly.

Presenting symptoms of HLH are due to the uncontrolled stimulation of macrophages and T cells, which causes overproduction of inflammatory cytokines, such as tumor necrosis factor α, IL-6, interferon-γ, and IL-1β, leading to an excessive inflammatory response (4). Secondary HLH can be due to several underlying conditions, such as infection, malignancy, or autoimmune disease (5).

Treatment of secondary HLH is not well defined, aside from aggressive management of the inciting condition. Directed agents, such as cyclosporine, etoposide, and corticosteroids, are used in treating primary disease, but their role in secondary disease is controversial. Sporadic case reports suggest success with different therapies, including antithymocyte globulin, monoclonal antibodies, and splenectomy. This patient improved with treatment of the primary infectious cause and supportive care.

Histoplasma capsulatum is a dimorphic fungus with a soil-based environmental reservoir. It is endemic in the Mississippi and Ohio river valleys. Patients with reduced cellular immunity (eg, AIDS, corticosteroid use, and extremes of age) are at risk for disseminated infection. Patients typically present with nonspecific systemic symptoms, including fever, malaise, anorexia, and weight loss. Cutaneous lesions or ulcerations, lymphadenopathy, or hepatosplenomegaly may also be present. Diagnosis is often delayed because of nonspecific symptoms and delayed identification of *Histoplasma* from clinical specimens.

A high level of awareness for HLH is key to diagnosing this fatal disease.

ACKNOWLEDGMENTS

Portions previously published in Thakur L, Iyer V. Rare case of histoplasmosis presenting with recurrent sepsis and hemophagocytic lymphohistiocytosis [abstract]. Crit Care Med. 2013 Dec;41(12 Suppl 1):A350. Used with permission.

REFERENCES

1. Janka G, zur Stadt U. Familial and acquired hemophagocytic lymphohistiocytosis. Hematology Am Soc Hematol Educ Program. 2005:82–8.

2. Demirkol D, Yildizdas D, Bayrakci B, Karapinar B, Kendirli T, Koroglu TF, et al; Turkish Secondary HLH/MAS Critical Care Study Group. Hyperferritinemia in the critically ill child with secondary hemophagocytic lymphohistiocytosis/sepsis/multiple organ dysfunction syndrome/macrophage activation syndrome: what is the treatment? Crit Care. 2012 Dec 12;16(2):R52.

3. Henter JI, Horne A, Arico M, Egeler RM, Filipovich AH, Imashuku S, et al. HLH-2004: diagnostic and therapeutic guidelines for hemophagocytic lymphohistiocytosis. Pediatr Blood Cancer. 2007 Feb;48(2):124–31.

4. Fujiwara F, Hibi S, Imashuku S. Hypercytokinemia in hemophagocytic syndrome. Am J Pediatr Hematol Oncol. 1993 Feb;15(1):92–8.

5. Janka G, Imashuku S, Elinder G, Schneider M, Henter JI. Infection- and malignancy-associated hemophagocytic syndromes: secondary hemophagocytic lymphohistiocytosis. Hematol Oncol Clin North Am. 1998 Apr;12(2):435–44.

A Curious Case of Abdominal Pain

PRAMOD K. GURU, MBBS,
ABBASALI AKHOUNDI, MD,
AND KIANOUSH B. KASHANI, MD

CASE PRESENTATION

A 64-year-old white man was admitted to the intensive care unit from the emergency department for management of abdominal pain associated with accelerated hypertension and acute kidney injury. The patient carried diagnoses of hypertension, hyperlipidemia, Graves disease, atrial fibrillation, and long-standing cardiomyopathy (most recent ejection fraction 50%). His presenting concerns were progressively worsening abdominal pain associated with nausea, vomiting, and diarrhea for the past 12 hours.

The patient was taking diltiazem, lisinopril, and warfarin. He reported multiple episodes of cardioversion in the past for a rapid ventricular rate due to atrial fibrillation, and he had undergone atrioventricular node ablation 5 days before this presentation. When he arrived at the emergency department, his blood pressure was 156/96 mm Hg and he rated his abdominal and flank pain as 7 out of 10 (on a scale from 0-10, where 10 is most severe). He reported that he had not had similar abdominal pain before; that he had not had dysuria, fever, renal colic, or prior surgery; and that he had not traveled recently or taken any new medication. His serum creatinine level increased from 0.9 to 1.6 mg/dL. He had leukocytosis (leukocytes 13.7×10^9/L), normal results from coagulation studies, and microscopic hematuria. After he received intravenous opioids and antihypertensives, his pain

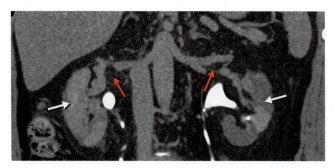

FIGURE 34.1. Renal Artery Dissection and Infarction. Abdominal computed tomographic coronal section shows bilateral renal artery dissection (red arrows) and infarction (white arrows). The absence of a smooth contour for the renal artery is evidenced by the contrast disruption.

subsided and his hypertension improved. Computed tomography of the abdomen showed bilateral renal and right external iliac artery dissection with multiple bilateral kidney infarcts (Figure 34.1).

Given the recent history of intravascular manipulation, the possibility of intervention-related dissection was entertained. However, because of the discontinuous and bilateral involvement of the renal arteries, the possibility of an inadvertent arterial puncture during the ablation and the subsequent dissection was dismissed. Results from serologic studies for vasculitides (antinuclear antibody, antineutrophil cytoplasmic autoantibody, C-reactive protein, and rheumatoid factor) and infections (hepatitis B and C viruses) were unremarkable. In the absence of other possible causes of dissection—with age, male sex, and hypertension as the risk factors—spontaneous dissection was diagnosed. During the remainder of his intensive care unit and hospital stays, the patient did not have recurrent pain, labile hypertension, or further worsening of renal function.

DISCUSSION

Spontaneous renal artery dissection is a rare cause of renovascular hypertension, but the renal artery is the most common site for dissection among the peripheral arteries (1). Since the mid 1980s and with the advent of radiologic procedures, renal artery dissections have been increasingly recognized (2). However, they are still uncommon, and the absolute number of cases reported in the medical literature is less than 300. Cases of bilateral renal artery dissection are even rarer and are reported in very limited case series (3). Abnormalities of the vasa vasorum and arterial dysplasia leading to spontaneous bleeding have been proposed as causes of dissection. However, the exact pathogenesis is unknown (4).

Association without proof of causality has been described with fibromuscular dysplasia (FMD), Ehlers-Danlos syndrome (EDS), malignant hypertension, atherosclerosis, antiphospholipid antibody syndrome, and polyarteritis nodosa (PAN) (1-3). Case reports of dissection after blunt trauma, severe exercise, cocaine abuse, and even shock wave lithotripsy have been described (1,2). In a case series of 17 patients (1), 4 patients had FMD, 4 had EDS, and 1 had PAN; the smoking rate did not differ from that of the general population; most affected patients were male and in their third or fourth decade of life; and, similar to the patient described above, these patients had abdominal pain, hematuria, and acute kidney injury as common presenting features. Other clinical features described are groin and testicular pain, fever, dysuria, nausea, and vomiting (2,4,5). For patients with risk factors who present with abdominal pain, the initial differential diagnosis and evaluation must exclude life-threatening and surgical emergencies, such as aortic dissection, mesenteric ischemia, and perforated bowel in addition to other benign and ominous causes of pain.

Common blood test findings are leukocytosis and elevated levels of creatinine and lactate dehydrogenase (1,4). Microscopic hematuria is the most common urinary abnormality. Angiography (either conventional or computed tomographic [CT]) is the diagnostic method of choice for most patients. Contrast-enhanced CT often shows renal infarction and can be used to help rule out most common renal emergencies, such as renal colic due to stones, renal abscess, pyelonephritis, renal vein thrombosis, and renal artery thromboembolism with infarction. Common radiologic findings are irregular caliber, double lumen, and bulging or aneurysm of the vessel (1,3). Although Doppler ultrasonography is inferior to CT angiography, it is noninvasive and avoids administration of a contrast agent.

Management is aimed at controlling symptoms, stabilizing the blood pressure, limiting infarction, and preventing recurrence (1,4,5). To avoid further renal injury, nonsteroidal anti-inflammatory drugs should not be used. Although a blood pressure target of 140/90 mm Hg has been acceptable to prevent further damage, the use of angiotensin-converting enzyme inhibitors and angiotensin receptor blockers should be avoided in the acute phase if the patient has a significantly elevated baseline creatinine (ie, >30% above the reference range) (1,2,4,5). The use of anticoagulation as a therapeutic option is controversial. Surgical interventions (radical or endovascular) are reserved for patients with worsening kidney function when medical therapy has failed.

Spontaneous renal artery dissection is an uncommon cause of abdominal pain and accelerated hypertension. It is associated with significant morbidity. A high level of awareness is needed for diagnosis.

REFERENCES

1. Afshinnia F, Sundaram B, Rao P, Stanley J, Bitzer M. Evaluation of characteristics, associations and clinical course of isolated spontaneous renal artery dissection. Nephrol Dial Transplant. 2013 Aug;28(8):2089–98. Epub 2013 Apr 5.

2. Edwards BS, Stanson AW, Holley KE, Sheps SG. Isolated renal artery dissection, presentation, evaluation, management, and pathology. Mayo Clin Proc. 1982 Sep;57(9):564–71.

3. Katz-Summercorn AC, Borg CM, Harris PL. Spontaneous renal artery dissection complicated by renal infarction: a case report and review of the literature. Int J Surg Case Rep. 2012;3(7):257–9. Epub 2012 Mar 20.

4. Lacombe M. Isolated spontaneous dissection of the renal artery. J Vasc Surg. 2001 Feb;33(2):385–91.

5. Ramamoorthy SL, Vasquez JC, Taft PM, McGinn RF, Hye RJ. Nonoperative management of acute spontaneous renal artery dissection. Ann Vasc Surg. 2002 Mar;16(2):157–62. Epub 2002 Feb 13.

Weakness in the Intensive Care Unit

CHRISTOPHER L. KRAMER, MD,
AND ALEJANDRO A. RABINSTEIN, MD

CASE PRESENTATION

A 52-year-old man presented to the medical intensive care unit (ICU) with hypoxic respiratory failure, pneumonia, acute respiratory distress syndrome, septic shock, encephalopathy, and acute renal failure. He had been intubated on admission through the emergency department, and mechanical ventilation with low tidal volumes and high positive end-expiratory pressure was initiated in the prone position. Ventilator synchrony was attained with a midazolam infusion and paralysis. Broad-spectrum antibiotics, aggressive fluid resuscitation, hydrocortisone, and norepinephrine were administered for septic shock. The renal failure progressed, and continuous renal replacement therapy was initiated. Despite an insulin drip, the patient's blood glucose level was difficult to control.

These therapies were continued for several days with resultant improvement in oxygenation and blood pressure. On day 6, paralysis and vasopressor support were discontinued. When sedation was stopped, the patient had diffuse limb weakness, globally decreased tone, and areflexia. Multiple attempts to wean him from mechanical ventilation were unsuccessful, despite significant improvement in his oxygenation and chest radiograph.

Nerve conduction studies (NCSs) showed severely reduced and prolonged compound muscle action potentials (CMAPs) and reduced sensory nerve action potentials (SNAPs) in multiple nerves. Mixed but predominantly small motor unit potentials were noted on electromyography (EMG). These findings were consistent with the diagnosis of critical illness neuromyopathy (CINM).

The patient subsequently underwent tracheostomy and was transferred to the respiratory care unit. He improved gradually with intensive physical therapy and was liberated from mechanical ventilation. After 11 days in the respiratory care unit, he was discharged to a rehabilitation facility, where he remained for 3 months before being discharged home.

DISCUSSION

CINM and the more recently proposed *ICU-acquired weakness* are diagnostic terms used to account for the common co-occurrence of both critical illness myopathy (CIM) and critical illness polyneuropathy (CIP) in weak, critically ill patients (1). The disease most commonly manifests as a flaccid quadriparesis, unsuccessful weaning from mechanical ventilation, and an inability to participate in physical therapy. CINM is extremely common—its incidence can approach 56% to 80% among patients with systemic inflammatory response syndrome (SIRS)/sepsis and multiorgan failure (2). Pathologically, CIP presents as a length-dependent sensorimotor polyneuropathy, and CIM as a myosin-dependent myopathy. NCSs and EMG are valuable in confirming the diagnosis and ruling out other potentially reversible causes of weakness. This is of great importance, because no specific treatment currently exists for CINM aside from aggressive risk factor modification and rehabilitation. Patients who have the disorder may have substantial disability (2).

Patients who have CIP or CIM present with various degrees of limb and diaphragm weakness. The diagnosis may be obscured initially by the confounding effects of coexistent encephalopathy or sedation and paralysis, and it may not become apparent until initiation of physical therapy or extubation failure (1). Clinical hallmarks of CIP include distal weakness and sensory loss and areflexia, with sparing of the facial and extraocular muscles. In contrast, weakness in CIM is typically proximal and can involve the face and, rarely, the extraocular muscles. No sensory loss occurs in CIM, and deep tendon reflexes are relatively preserved. However, CIM and CIP rarely occur in isolation and their coexistence is actually more common (1,2).

While the presence and severity of SIRS/sepsis and multiorgan failure are the most prominent risk factors for CINM, other risk factors associated with the disorder include prolonged mechanical ventilation and ICU stay, corticosteroid administration, hyperglycemia, renal failure, neuromuscular junction blocking agent use, and poor nutritional status (2). The pathologic result in CIP is a length-dependent axonal sensorimotor polyneuropathy. In CIM, myosin loss is the pathologic hallmark. Functionally, a sodium channelopathy in CIM results in inexcitable muscle tissue (1).

Treatment options for CINM are currently limited, so the exclusion of other causes of weakness, including a preexisting neuromuscular disorder, is paramount. Detailed history and physical examination are essential to localize the problem. If a central neurologic cause of the weakness is suspected, neuroimaging may be indicated. Laboratory studies including an electrolyte panel with magnesium, calcium, and phosphorus levels should be used to rule out metabolic causes of weakness. Serum creatine kinase levels are usually normal or mildly elevated in CINM, except for a rare necrotizing form. Significant elevation should prompt further investigation into other forms of myopathies, including inflammatory myopathies, toxic myopathies, muscular dystrophy, and acid maltase deficiency (1).

NCSs and EMG are extremely helpful for confirming the diagnosis of CINM and excluding other illnesses. Repetitive nerve stimulation is normal in CINM, but it can be used to detect neuromuscular transmission failure, such as that caused by prolonged blockade with paralytics and myasthenia gravis. CMAPs are typically reduced and prolonged, and SNAPs can be diminished in CINM (3). Nerve conduction velocity, however, is relatively preserved, and slowing can indicate demyelinating pathology such as Guillain-Barré syndrome. Motor units on EMG can vary from large to small depending on the relative contribution of CIM and CIP. The absence of widespread fasciculations can help rule out amyotrophic lateral sclerosis (1).

Direct muscle stimulation has been used to differentiate CIM from CIP (muscle contracts in CIP but not in CIM) (1); however, this may be difficult to perform and interpret in practice. Cerebrospinal fluid results are normal in CINM, and lumbar puncture is not routinely necessary unless there is clinical suspicion of an alternative diagnosis. Muscle ultrasonography has recently been shown to be a promising aid in the diagnosis of CINM (4). Muscle and nerve biopsy can be used to establish a definitive diagnosis but is rarely used in clinical practice.

There is no specific treatment for CINM. Thus, aggressive risk factor management is essential to reduce its incidence. A recent Cochrane meta-analysis

(5) found an association between intensive insulin therapy and a reduction in the incidence of CINM, duration of mechanical ventilation, and 180-day mortality, albeit with a higher incidence of hypoglycemic events. Early rehabilitation in CINM was associated with shorter duration of mechanical ventilation, although there was no effect on ICU length of stay.

Mortality is high among patients with sepsis and CINM, but survivors improve gradually and may achieve good functional recovery. Although evidence is not uniform, CIM may carry a better prognosis than CIP (2).

REFERENCES

1. Bolton CF. Neuromuscular manifestations of critical illness. Muscle Nerve. 2005 Aug;32(2):140–63.

2. Latronico N, Bolton CF. Critical illness polyneuropathy and myopathy: a major cause of muscle weakness and paralysis. Lancet Neurol. 2011 Oct;10(10):931–41.

3. Goodman BP, Harper CM, Boon AJ. Prolonged compound muscle action potential duration in critical illness myopathy. Muscle Nerve. 2009 Dec;40(6):1040–2.

4. Grimm A, Teschner U, Porzelius C, Ludewig K, Zielske J, Witte OW, et al. Muscle ultrasound for early assessment of critical illness neuromyopathy in severe sepsis. Crit Care. 2013 Oct 7;17(5):R227.

5. Hermans G, De Jonghe B, Bruyninckx F, Van den Berghe G. Interventions for preventing critical illness polyneuropathy and critical illness myopathy. Cochrane Database Syst Rev. 2014 Jan 30;1:CD006832.

Altered Mental Status and Rigidity

CHRISTOPHER L. KRAMER, MD, AND ALEJANDRO A. RABINSTEIN, MD

CASE PRESENTATION

A 56-year-old woman with a history of schizophrenia presented to the emergency department after being found on the floor at home by her husband. She was severely encephalopathic and rigid. He had noticed that she had become increasingly confused over the preceding 2 days. Her medication for schizophrenia had been switched 1 month ago from olanzapine 10 mg daily to risperidone 6 mg daily, and she had tolerated the medication without any significant side effects.

On admission the patient was afebrile but tachycardic and hypertense. Her left leg was markedly edematous and tense with absent dorsalis pedis and tibial artery pulses. Red urine was noted in the Foley catheter bag. Neurologically, she was mute but able to track objects and intermittently follow commands. Diffuse fine tremors and waxy flexibility were noted in addition to marked axial and bilateral rigidity in her arms and legs. Laboratory test results showed moderate leukocytosis, hyponatremia with normal serum osmolality, markedly elevated creatine kinase (CK) level (17,637 U/L), normal creatinine concentration, myoglobinuria, and lactate 0.3 mmol/L. Findings on computed tomography of the head and cervical spine were unremarkable. The patient was subsequently admitted to the medical intensive care unit with a suspected diagnosis of neuroleptic malignant syndrome (NMS) with rhabdomyolysis and compartment syndrome of the left leg.

Risperidone was immediately discontinued, and she was given intravenous dantrolene 60 mg every 4 hours. She was hydrated aggressively and given bicarbonate to alkalinize the urine, which successfully prevented the development of acute tubular necrosis related to the rhabdomyolysis with myoglobinuria. Compartment syndrome of her left lower extremity prompted urgent surgical evaluation, and she was quickly taken to the operating room for a fasciotomy.

Her rigidity and encephalopathy improved over the following days, and the patient was transitioned to oral bromocriptine 2.5 mg 3 times daily for 10 days. She had minor fevers and fluctuations in blood pressure and heart rate that did not require treatment. Her CK slowly normalized. Her hyponatremia, which was discovered to be related to psychogenic polydipsia, was slowly corrected. She experienced gradual and complete clinical recovery.

DISCUSSION

NMS is a rare but potentially lethal neurologic emergency associated with depletion of central nervous system dopamine from the use of antipsychotic medications or the sudden withdrawal of dopaminergic agents. Cardinal clinical features of the disorder include motor symptoms (predominantly rigidity), hypokinetic encephalopathy, hyperthermia, and dysautonomia. The rigidity can cause severe elevations in serum CK and rhabdomyolysis. Prompt recognition of the disorder and withdrawal of the offending antidopaminergic agent, supportive care of systemic manifestations such as rhabdomyolysis and autonomic instability, and implementation of treatment with bromocriptine or dantrolene (or both) can improve the outcome (1).

NMS is estimated to occur in 0.07% to 2.2% of all patients treated with antipsychotic medications (2). It is associated with a mortality rate of 5% to 20%, which is strongly affected by the presence and severity of dysautonomia and associated nonneurologic comorbidities. Traditionally related to the use of typical antipsychotics, the condition may be precipitated by atypical antiemetics (eg, prochlorperazine, droperidol, and metoclopramide) and the sudden withdrawal of dopaminergic agents.

Proposed risk factors for the development of NMS include a previous history of NMS, use of high doses of neuroleptics, a recent large increase in a neuroleptic dose, parenteral administration of antipsychotics, the use of 2 or more neuroleptics, and concomitant lithium use. It occurs most commonly within the first

TABLE 36.1. **Differential Diagnosis of Neuroleptic Malignant Syndrome and Differentiating Clinical Features**

Syndrome	Differentiating Clinical Features
Neuroleptic malignant syndrome	Normal pupils, lead pipe rigidity, hypokinesis, depressed reflexes, stupor, mutism, possible catatonic features, dysautonomia (may be severe)
Serotonin syndrome	Mydriasis, hyperkinesis and agitation, hyperreflexia and rigidity most prominent in the legs, clonus, diarrhea
Anticholinergic toxicity	Mydriasis, erythematous and dry mucosa, constipation, urinary retention, absence of paroxysmal dysautonomia, agitation
Malignant hyperthermia	Normal pupils, extreme hyperthermia, mottled mucosa, "rigor mortis" rigidity, hyporeflexia, use of inhalational anesthetic or succinylcholine
Paroxysmal sympathetic hyperactivity	Episodic mydriasis, diaphoresis, tachycardia, hypertension, fever, dystonic posturing associated with significant central nervous system injury
Sympathomimetic toxicity	Mydriasis, diaphoresis, significant tachycardia, less hyperthermia, agitation
Malignant catatonia	Symptoms occur before neuroleptic administration; behavioral changes occur weeks before syndrome; choreiform movements, waxy flexibility, posturing

2 weeks of oral neuroleptic therapy (1), yet NMS can occur after a single dose of a neuroleptic or after treatment with the same agent at the same dose for many years.

NMS usually develops over 24 to 72 hours, and up to 82% of patients present with a partial syndrome. The presenting symptom in 70% of patients is altered mental status (3). Therefore, the initial presentation of NMS may be nonspecific, and a high level of awareness may be necessary for at-risk patients. The initial differential diagnosis may be broad (Table 36.1).

Lead pipe rigidity is the most common motor manifestation of NMS; however, tremor, bradykinesia or akinesia, dystonia, and dyskinesias can also be seen. Hyperthermia is commonly present and can be severe (>41°C). Autonomic symptoms include respiratory irregularities, blood pressure fluctuations, diaphoresis, and cardiac arrhythmias. Important nonneurologic comorbidities include rhabdomyolysis (and rarely compartment syndrome [4]), associated renal failure, electrolyte abnormalities, metabolic acidosis, deep vein thrombosis, and pulmonary embolism (1).

The most important aspect of treating NMS is removal of the offending agent and avoidance of antidopaminergic agents. Supportive treatment includes aggressively regulating temperature, monitoring for arrhythmias, and treating arrhythmias. Blood pressure should be maintained carefully, preferably with fluids or short-acting vasodilators to avoid overshooting. Intubation and mechanical ventilation may be required for patients with respiratory failure from inadequate tidal volume due to severe chest wall rigidity and autonomic failure (1). Treatment of rhabdomyolysis with high volumes of crystalloid fluids and urine alkalization, if necessary, is the paramount step to prevent or treat associated renal failure from myoglobinuria. Deep vein thrombosis prophylaxis is important because rigidity and immobility may increase the risk of clot formation (1).

Treatment with bromocriptine, a central dopamine agonist, has been speculated to improve outcomes in NMS, although study bias limits definitive proof of efficacy. If treatment is initiated, it should continue for at least 10 days after symptom resolution (longer with depot agents) and should be followed by tapered dosing. Dantrolene, a skeletal muscle relaxant, can be added in more severe cases to reduce fever and muscle rigidity (1). Major side effects include hepatotoxicity (with dantrolene) and hypotension (with bromocriptine). For refractory cases, electroconvulsive therapy has also been used to treat NMS. Treatment has been associated with reduced time to recovery and decreased mortality (5), although the efficacy of this therapy has not been confirmed in large studies. Reinstitution of a neuroleptic, if necessary, should wait until at least 2 weeks after symptom resolution, and patients should begin receiving a lower dose of antipsychotics and be monitored closely for reemergence of symptoms.

REFERENCES

1. Bhanushali MJ, Tuite PJ. The evaluation and management of patients with neuroleptic malignant syndrome. Neurol Clin. 2004 May;22(2):389–411.

2. Adnet P, Lestavel P, Krivosic-Horber R. Neuroleptic malignant syndrome. Br J Anaesth. 2000 Jul;85(1):129–35.

3. Velamoor VR, Norman RM, Caroff SN, Mann SC, Sullivan KA, Antelo RE. Progression of symptoms in neuroleptic malignant syndrome. J Nerv Ment Dis. 1994 Mar;182(3):168–73.

4. Schneider JM, Roger DJ, Uhl RL. Bilateral forearm compartment syndromes resulting from neuroleptic malignant syndrome. J Hand Surg Am. 1996 Mar;21(2):287–9.

5. Davis JM, Janicak PG, Sakkas P, Gilmore C, Wang Z. Electroconvulsive therapy in the treatment of the neuroleptic malignant syndrome. Convuls Ther. 1991;7(2):111–120.

Overdose

ARJUN GUPTA, MBBS, AND SAHIL KHANNA, MBBS

CASE PRESENTATION

A 29-year-old man presented to the emergency department with nausea and acute-onset right upper quadrant abdominal pain of 1 day's duration. The medical history included chronic alcoholic pancreatitis and distal pancreatectomy, bipolar disorder, seizure disorder, and polysubstance abuse; current medications included pancrelipase, escitalopram, and oxcarbazepine. He reported no alcohol or drug abuse. He was hypotensive (blood pressure 80/30 mm Hg) and tachycardic but afebrile. On physical examination, the patient was jaundiced, irritable, and malnourished with abdominal tenderness but no stigmata of chronic liver disease. Laboratory evaluation showed anion gap metabolic acidosis; elevated lactate, white blood cell count (15×10^9/L), and creatinine; international normalized ratio (INR) 4.3; bilirubin 1.5 mg/dL; aspartate aminotransferase (AST) 1,350 U/L and alanine aminotransferase (ALT) 1,240 U/L; glucose 45 mg/dL; and lipase within the reference range. Computed tomography (CT) of the abdomen to rule out an acute process showed ileus of the small bowel with unremarkable liver anatomy. The patient was hydrated with normal saline with added dextrose; he was given intravenous vancomycin and piperacillin-tazobactam and was admitted to the medical intensive care unit. The differential diagnosis included acute liver failure secondary to sepsis, shock liver, drug reaction or toxicity, viral hepatitis, and autoimmune hepatitis.

The patient's condition rapidly deteriorated over the next 6 hours, and he became drowsy and disoriented to time and place, with worsening jaundice. He was intubated and sedated for airway protection given his comatose state. Laboratory evaluation showed INR 6.1 (which had increased even after administration of fresh frozen plasma and vitamin K), AST 6,500 U/L, ALT 3,350 U/L, bilirubin 42 mg/dL, thrombocytopenia (platelets 29×10^9/L), and serum ammonia 193 mcmol/L. Because sepsis was a concern, antimicrobial coverage was expanded to include amphotericin B, acyclovir, levofloxacin, and doxycycline. Results from CT of the head, blood and urine cultures, chest radiography, viral hepatitis markers, and urine toxicology screening were negative except for threshold positivity for opiates. Serum monohydroxy carbamazepine levels were within the therapeutic range. The serum acetaminophen level measured 3 hours after presentation was elevated (46 mcg/mL) (the therapeutic range varies with time since ingestion, but the levels decrease sharply after peaking at 4 hours); serum salicylate and osmolal gap values were normal. Levels of autoimmune markers and serum ceruloplasmin were normal. Ultrasonography of the abdomen showed normal liver echotexture and patent vasculature. Tests for herpesviruses, fungal diseases, and tick-borne illness were also negative.

A diagnosis of acute liver failure secondary to acetaminophen ingestion was made, and a 72-hour protocol of *N*-acetylcysteine (NAC) was initiated with a loading dose of 140 mg/kg. A family member later reported that 75 tablets of oxycodone-acetaminophen (5 mg-325 mg), equivalent to more than 24 g of acetaminophen, were missing since an unconfirmed time.

Rifaximin and lactulose were administered for hepatic encephalopathy, and an intracranial pressure monitor showed pressures in the low-normal range except for 1 spike to 28 mm Hg that was managed satisfactorily with a single bolus dose of mannitol. Liver transplant was considered, and the patient was treated with the molecular adsorbent recirculating system (MARS; Gambro) for 2 days. He showed dramatic clinical improvement after undergoing that treatment and receiving NAC therapy, with a rapid return to baseline neurologic status, and his liver enzymes returned to baseline levels in 6 days. He was discharged after psychiatric consultation.

DISCUSSION

Acetaminophen overdose is the most common medication poisoning reported to US poison control centers and is the most common cause of acute liver failure in the western world (1). Acetaminophen is a component of several over-the-counter and prescription medications. Overdose can be intentional or accidental, and it should be considered in the differential diagnosis of markedly elevated liver enzymes. Management includes early recognition, supportive management, removal of unabsorbed medication, prompt antidote administration, and referral to a liver transplant center (1).

When patients present with liver enzyme levels greater than 1,000 U/L, the differential diagnosis includes acute viral infections, ischemia, acetaminophen and other drug or toxin poisoning, and rarely autoimmune hepatitis, Wilson disease, and acute fatty liver of pregnancy. A targeted history and serum acetaminophen level should be obtained for all patients who have acute liver failure with severe transaminitis (>1,000 U/L) and possible acetaminophen intake. Acetaminophen toxicity is dose-dependent and rarely occurs at ingestion of less than 4 g daily, although the threshold for toxicity can be lower because of age, poor nutritional status, chronic liver disease, coingestions, alcohol intake, and an induced hepatic cytochrome P450 system.

Symptoms can be subtle in the first 24 hours, with only nausea, vomiting, and malaise (stage 1). Changes during the next 72 hours are dramatic, with worsening liver dysfunction and multiorgan failure followed by paradoxical initial clinical improvement (stages 2 and 3). Stage 4, the recovery phase for patients who survive, is usually complete in 1 to 2 weeks.

Knowing the time of acetaminophen ingestion is important for following symptoms, interpreting drug levels, and devising appropriate management. Activated charcoal may be used in an attempt to remove unabsorbed drug in the first 4 hours if the patient is conscious. A nomogram can be used to decide about the need for NAC therapy if serum acetaminophen levels are measured from 4 to 24 hours after ingestion. The nomogram is not useful if the time of ingestion is unknown, if more than 24 hours has passed since ingestion, or if the patient took multiple oral doses. An early referral to a liver transplant center should be considered if there is evidence of worsening synthetic dysfunction and encephalopathy, but there are no refined criteria for when to proceed (2).

The patient described above was managed appropriately with initial stabilization and admission to the intensive care unit for management of acute liver failure. The high levels of transaminases (>1,000 U/L) helped to narrow the differential diagnosis considerably and raised a concern for acetaminophen toxicity.

Broad-spectrum antimicrobial therapy was initiated because the patient's presentation fulfilled the criteria for systemic inflammatory response syndrome; antimicrobial therapy was stopped only after all culture and microbiological results were negative. Activated charcoal was not administered because the time since ingestion was likely much greater than 4 hours. Although the serum acetaminophen level was elevated, it was impossible to interpret because the time since ingestion was unknown. Although NAC works best if administered within 8 hours after ingestion, it is beneficial at any time and should be given when overdose is a concern (3). The patient described above had a history of ingestion, elevated transaminase levels, and liver failure.

REFERENCES

1. Lee WM, Squires RH Jr, Nyberg SL, Doo E, Hoofnagle JH. Acute liver failure: summary of a workshop. Hepatology. 2008 Apr;47(4):1401–15.
2. Brok J, Buckley N, Gluud C. Interventions for paracetamol (acetaminophen) overdose. Cochrane Database Syst Rev. 2006 Apr 19;(2):CD003328.
3. Iqbal M, Cash WJ, Sarwar S, McCormick PA. Paracetamol overdose: the liver unit perspective. Ir J Med Sci. 2012 Sep;181(3):439–43. Epub 2011 Nov 10.

An Unusual Encephalopathy

RUDY M. TEDJA, DO,
AND TENG MOUA, MD

CASE PRESENTATION

A 48-year-old man was admitted for increased abdominal and lower extremity swelling. He was an active alcoholic, with his latest consumption on the day before admission. He had a known history of alcoholic cirrhosis, with a current Model for End-Stage Liver Disease (MELD) score of 21, and associated esophageal varices. No ascites was detected on abdominal ultrasonography. On hospital day 2, hematemesis and hypotension developed, for which he was transferred to the medical intensive care unit (ICU) for emergent esophagogastroduodenoscopy (EGD). He was subsequently intubated for airway protection. Etomidate was used for intubation, and propofol and fentanyl were used for moderate sedation. During endoscopy, multiple esophageal varices larger than 5 mm were noted in the middle third and lower third of the esophagus, all of which were subsequently banded. Intravenous octreotide and a proton pump inhibitor were started. Multiple blood product transfusions were also given.

The patient was hemodynamically stable after the procedure and was weaned from sedation; however, after several hours, he was unarousable to sternal rub. On physical examination, he was found to be in decerebrate posturing with lower extremity rigidity, hyperreflexia, myoclonus, and a positive Babinski sign in the left foot. Computed tomography (CT) of the head showed no intracranial hemorrhage or cerebral edema. An electroencephalogram showed diffuse, severe,

generalized slowing without evidence of epileptiform discharge. No electrolyte abnormalities were noted. Serum creatinine and blood glucose values were
within the reference ranges. The ammonia level was elevated (105 mcmol/L).
The patient was febrile (38.2°C). Blood cultures were positive for *Streptococcus
mitis*. Ceftriaxone therapy was initiated with subsequent negative blood cultures.
Lactulose therapy was initiated through a nasogastric tube; however, aggressive
therapy with maximal dosing failed to produce bowel movements. A lactulose
enema was administered. After 24 hours, the patient remained unresponsive,
although his decerebrate posturing with rigidity improved. A gastroenterologist
recommended a transjugular intrahepatic portosystemic shunt (TIPS) given the
high risk of variceal rebleeding. Aggressive lactulose therapy was continued until
ICU day 7, when the patient's mental status began to improve. He was eventually
extubated without complication on ICU day 8.

DISCUSSION

Hepatic encephalopathy is not an uncommon neuropsychiatric abnormality in
patients with liver dysfunction, particularly advanced cirrhosis. It results from
portosystemic venous shunting, and presentation varies from an abnormal sleep
pattern to somnolence and deep coma. Traditionally, the severity of hepatic
encephalopathy has been categorized into 4 major grades (1-4) denoting worsening levels of consciousness and responsiveness. Grade 1 manifests as a mild
change in cognitive behavior; grade 2 as lethargy and moderate confusion; grade
3 as marked confusion with incoherent speech and hypersomnolence upon
awakening to examination; and grade 4 as coma (1). Neuromotor impairment
in severe hepatic encephalopathy also varies from asterixis to bradykinesia and
hyperreflexia. In general, neurologic manifestations are symmetric, although they
may be focal.

It is rare to find decerebrate or decorticate posturing, although this has been
described in the literature (2,3). Generally, both decerebrate and decorticate posturing result from an ischemic or anatomical insult to areas of the brain below
the cortex and usually indicate a more ominous, focally injurious, and irreversible
process. Decerebrate posturing usually occurs in patients with grade 4 encephalopathy, suggesting that the patient is more critically ill and has a worse prognosis.

However, the pathophysiology of such findings in overt hepatic encephalopathy is unknown. A prior study suggests a possible predilection for brainstem

structures in patients with hepatic encephalopathy, although this assumption is theoretical and requires further study (4). The patient described above had transient decerebrate posturing along with a focal Babinski sign on the left that resolved within 24 hours. Immediate CT of the head did not show intracranial abnormalities. When confronted with posturing, concerning structural abnormalities should be ruled out immediately by appropriate imaging studies because prompt surgical and medical attention may be lifesaving. The patient described above recovered completely after 5 days of supportive therapy. The cause of hepatic encephalopathy was likely multifactorial given the acute infection, the variceal hemorrhage, and the subsequent TIPS procedure.

Decerebrate posturing is uncommon in patients with cirrhosis and hepatic encephalopathy. Assessing for ischemic or structural intracranial abnormalities should be pursued immediately because prompt surgical and medical therapy specifically targeted to secondary causes may be lifesaving. The pathophysiology of decerebrate posturing in patients with hepatic encephalopathy is unknown, although it appears to be reversible with aggressive management of the underlying encephalopathy.

REFERENCES

1. Ferenci P, Lockwood A, Mullen K, Tarter R, Weissenborn K, Blei AT. Hepatic encephalopathy: definition, nomenclature, diagnosis, and quantification: final report of the working party at the 11th World Congresses of Gastroenterology, Vienna, 1998. Hepatology. 2002 Mar;35(3):716–21.

2. Wehbe E, Saad D, Delgado F, Ta H, Antoun SA. Reversible hepatic decerebration: a case report and review of the literature. Eur J Gastroenterol Hepatol. 2010 Jun;22(6):759–60.

3. Conomy JP, Swash M. Reversible decerebrate and decorticate postures in hepatic coma. N Engl J Med. 1968 Apr 18;278(16):876–9.

4. Juneja I, Yovic A. Hepatic decerebration. Neurology. 1972 May;22(5):537–9.

Brain Death

DEREDDI RAJA S. REDDY, MD,
SUDHIR V. DATAR, MBBS,
AND EELCO F. M. WIJDICKS, MD, PhD

CASE PRESENTATION

A 46-year-old woman was admitted to the intensive care unit after 15 minutes of cardiopulmonary resuscitation for out-of-hospital pulseless electrical activity arrest. Her background history was significant for diabetes mellitus, end-stage renal disease treated with hemodialysis, and 3-vessel coronary artery bypass graft surgery. On arrival she had a core temperature of 33°C, and she was acidemic (pH 6.8) and hyperkalemic (potassium 6.9 mmol/L). She underwent emergent dialysis to correct the acidosis and hyperkalemia. To maintain a systolic blood pressure of more than 100 mm Hg, she was given an epinephrine and dobutamine infusion. She did not receive any sedatives. Computed tomography of the brain showed features consistent with diffuse hypoxic ischemic injury: loss of differentiation between gray matter and white matter and diffuse cerebral edema with complete effacement of the sulci and basal cisterns. The next morning, in the absence of any confounding circumstances, the patient's neurologic examination showed absent brainstem reflexes (absent pupillary light reflex, corneal reflex, oculocephalic reflex, cold caloric reflex, gag reflex, and cough reflex) and no motor response to pain. An apnea test was attempted after the patient received preoxygenation with 100% fraction of inspired oxygen. Oxygen was delivered at 6 L/min through a small cannula into the endotracheal tube at the level of the carina after she was disconnected from the ventilator. Her baseline Pco_2 was 37 mm Hg and her temperature was 37°C. After 8 minutes of the apnea test, her Pco_2 increased to 61 mm Hg, with no spontaneous breathing. She met the criteria for brain death.

DISCUSSION

Deeply comatose patients who lose all clinical signs of brain function (including brainstem function) because of a major destructive lesion should be clearly distinguished from patients with other comatose states. When an untreatable catastrophic neurologic structural injury has been proved, irreversibility is determined by absent motor responses, loss of all brainstem reflexes, and apnea after a carbon dioxide challenge (1). Malignant ischemic infarction, intracerebral hemorrhage, severe traumatic brain injury, and aneurysmal subarachnoid hemorrhage are some of the common causes (2). Most patients do not become brain-dead after such an injury, and therefore a careful examination into possible confounders is needed. In clinical practice, neurologists, neurosurgeons, and intensivists are often asked to make that determination (3). The American Academy of Neurology has issued guidelines for determining brain death that were based on a thorough review of the existing evidence (1).

Clinical examination is the standard for determining brain death, and the apnea test forms a crucial component. However, before proceeding with brain death examination, the clinician must verify that 1) the causative factor is irreversible and 2) all confounding factors are eliminated (3) (Box 39.1).

If suspicion of central nervous system depression due to drugs or drug paralytics is suspected, adequate time should be allowed (about 5 half-lives) for the clearance of the drug (if the patient has normal hepatic and renal function). Serum and urine drug screening should be considered. Drug metabolism may be delayed considerably by prior use of therapeutic hypothermia and by liver function abnormalities that are associated with hypotension. All electrolyte, acid-base, and endocrine disturbances known to affect the level of consciousness must be corrected. To perform a reliable neurologic examination, the patient's temperature should be warmer than 36°C and systolic blood pressure should be greater than 100 mm Hg. The clinical examination should show lack of all responsiveness. A noxious stimulus should not produce any motor response, eye opening, or eye movements except for occasional reflex responses mediated by the spinal cord.

BOX 39.1.
CHECKLIST FOR DETERMINING BRAIN DEATH

Prerequisites (all must be checked)

Coma—irreversible and cause known

Neuroimaging explains coma

CNS-depressant drug effect absent (if indicated, toxicology screen; if barbiturates have been given, serum level <10 mcg/mL)

No evidence of residual paralytics (electrical stimulation if paralytics were used)

Absence of severe acid-base, electrolyte, or endocrine abnormality

Normothermia or mild hypothermia (core temperature >36°C)

Systolic blood pressure ≥100 mm Hg

No spontaneous respirations

Examination (all must be checked)

Pupils nonreactive to bright light

Corneal reflex absent

Oculocephalic reflex absent (tested only if cervical spine integrity is ensured)

Oculovestibular reflex absent

No facial movement to noxious stimuli at supraorbital nerve or temporomandibular joint

Gag reflex absent

Cough reflex absent with tracheal suctioning

Absence of motor response to noxious stimuli in all 4 limbs (spinally mediated reflexes are permissible)

Apnea testing (all must be checked)

Patient is hemodynamically stable

Ventilator is adjusted to provide normocapnia ($Paco_2$ 34-45 mm Hg)

Patient has been preoxygenated with 100% Fio_2 for >10 min to Pao_2 >200 mm Hg

Patient is well oxygenated with a PEEP of 5 cm H_2O

Provide oxygen through a suction catheter to the level of the carina at 6 L/min or attach a T-piece with CPAP at 10 cm H_2O

Disconnect ventilator

Spontaneous respirations absent

Arterial blood gas drawn at 8-10 min; patient reconnected to ventilator

Pco_2 ≥60 mm Hg, or a 20–mm Hg increase from normal baseline value

or

Apnea test aborted

Ancillary testing (only 1 needs to be performed; to be ordered only if clinical examination cannot be fully performed because of patient factors, or if apnea testing is inconclusive or aborted)

Cerebral angiography

Technetium Tc 99m–hexamethylpropylemeamine oxime single-photon emission computed tomography

Electroencephalography

Transcranial Doppler ultrasonography

Abbreviations: CNS, central nervous system; CPAP, continuous positive airway pressure; FIO_2, fraction of inspired oxygen; PEEP, positive end-expiratory pressure.

Adapted from Wijdicks et al (1). Used with permission.

Examination of the brainstem reflexes should show an absence of the pupillary light reflex, corneal reflex, oculocephalic reflex, and oculovestibular reflexes (inserting cold water into both ears); an absence of facial movements to noxious stimuli; and an absence of gag and cough reflexes. The oculocephalic reflex cannot be tested if a cervical spine injury is suspected, and blood or cerumen in the ear canal can interfere with oculovestibular reflexes when cold water does not reach the eardrum. The cough reflex can be reliably tested by examining the cough response to tracheal suctioning. The catheter should be inserted into the trachea and advanced to the level of the carina followed by 1 or 2 suctioning passes (1). The rationale behind doing an apnea test is to induce metabolic acidosis and cerebrospinal fluid acidosis to stimulate the chemoreceptors in the medulla oblongata. In the United States, the threshold for establishing the absence of a respiratory drive has been set at a $Paco_2$ of 60 mm Hg or a value that is 20 mm Hg higher than the normal baseline value.

After the prerequisites are met and confounders are excluded, the clinician can proceed to the apnea test and use the oxygen-diffusion method, which remains a preferred method and is very simple (4).

REFERENCES

1. Wijdicks EF, Varelas PN, Gronseth GS, Greer DM; American Academy of Neurology. Evidence-based guideline update: determining brain death in adults: report of the Quality

Standards Subcommittee of the American Academy of Neurology. Neurology. 2010 Jun 8;74(23):1911–8.

2. Wijdicks EF. The diagnosis of brain death. N Engl J Med. 2001 Apr 19;344(16):1215–21.

3. Wijdicks EFM. Brain death, 2nd ed. Oxford (UK): Oxford University Press; c2011.

4. Datar S, Fugate J, Rabinstein A, Couillard P, Wijdicks EF. Completing the apnea test: decline in complications. Neurocrit Care. 2014 Dec;21(3):392–6.

Use of Extracorporeal Membrane Oxygenation for Acute Respiratory Distress Syndrome

KELLY A. CAWCUTT, MD,
CRAIG E. DANIELS, MD,
AND GREGORY J. SCHEARS, MD

CASE PRESENTATION

A 31-year-old man presented to another medical facility with a 1-week history of shortness of breath, nonproductive cough, headaches, chills, and malaise. He reportedly had no laboratory testing or imaging evaluation, and he was given an empirical diagnosis of carbon monoxide poisoning and was then dismissed. The following day, after driving several hours in the car to visit a friend, he became acutely dyspneic and was taken to a local emergency department. He was noted to have hypoxic respiratory failure and bradycardia. Chest radiography was significant for diffuse bilateral infiltrates. He was intubated and, during transfer to a local facility with a medical intensive care unit, he was noted to be severely hypoxic (peripheral oxygen saturation about 50%) and acidemic (arterial blood gas pH 6.9), and he subsequently had a cardiac arrest with return of spontaneous circulation after 8 to 12 minutes of advanced cardiac life support.

Upon arrival at the receiving hospital, he remained hypoxic despite aggressive management. Echocardiography showed low-normal left ventricular systolic function with an ejection fraction of 50% to 55%, moderate right ventricular hypokinesis, elevated right atrial pressure 20 mm Hg, no intracardiac shunts, and no significant valve disease. After the cardiac evaluation did not show a reversible cardiac cause of his refractory hypoxemia, the patient underwent extracorporeal membrane oxygenation (ECMO) cannulation with a bicaval, dual-lumen ECMO catheter placed in the right internal jugular vein to allow for initiation of veno-venous (VV) ECMO. He was then transferred to a regional ECMO center for further management.

On admission to the ECMO center, he was noted to have myxedema coma signs, including hypothermia, bradycardia, pretibial and periorbital edema, and decreased eyebrow and body hair. He was given intravenous thyroid hormone and steroid replacement therapy. Further, he had new, severe left ventricular dysfunction with an ejection fraction of 22%, and it was noted that the ECMO catheter was malpositioned, with the cannula in the right ventricle. Therefore, in the operating room, the ECMO was transitioned from VV ECMO to venoarterial (VA) ECMO.

An extensive evaluation, including clinical examination, imaging, and laboratory evaluation, was completed to determine the underlying cause of his severe, hypoxic respiratory failure and acute respiratory distress syndrome (ARDS). Upon receipt and review of the patient's medical records, the medical team discovered that the patient had a past medical history of thyroid ablation, with a history of nonadherence to hormone replacement therapy; this information explained his myxedema coma. Ultimately, he was given a diagnosis of *Legionella* pneumonia, ARDS, *Legionella* bloodstream infection, myxedema coma, and acute kidney injury requiring renal replacement therapy.

The patient continued to receive ECMO for 21 days. He was treated with supportive care, thyroid replacement therapy, and 21 days of levofloxacin for *Legionella* pneumonia and *Legionella* bloodstream infection. After decannulation from the ECMO circuitry and liberation from mechanical ventilation with his decreased need for sedative or hypnotic agents, the patient was noted to have significant encephalopathy. No reversible cause was documented and, with the assistance of a neurologist's evaluation, he was given the diagnosis of anoxic brain injury.

The patient was discharged to an acute rehabilitation facility from the hospital approximately 55 days after admission. At discharge, he no longer required dialysis and could ambulate independently.

DISCUSSION

Extracorporeal life support (ECLS) is intended to temporarily provide mechanical cardiopulmonary support. ECMO is the most common ECLS technology used outside the operating room, and it can be used to support patients for days to weeks. For neonates and children, ECMO has shown ample evidence of benefit and is widely accepted. Historically, this has not been the case for adults, but in recent years the use of ECMO has increased for adult patients with acute respiratory failure, including ARDS (1,2). Several factors have contributed to this increased use of ECMO in adults with ARDS, including improved biocompatibility of the circuitry, which minimizes adverse events; clinical trial data, which provide evidence of a survival benefit (Conventional Ventilation or ECMO for Severe Adult Respiratory Failure [CESAR] trial); clinical experience showing improved outcomes during the 2009 pandemic with the H1N1 influenza virus; and decreased use of high-frequency oscillation as an alternative rescue strategy because trials have shown evidence of harm (Oscillation for ARDS Treated Early [OSCILLATE] trial; Oscillation in ARDS [OSCAR] study) (3).

The increasing use of ECMO for adults with acute respiratory failure necessitates that all intensivists have a basic understanding of the indications, complications, and current outcomes for patients. Intensivists must be prepared to participate in informed discussions with families, to provide appropriate and timely care, and to transfer patients who may benefit from ECMO.

The patient described above is an example of a patient with acute respiratory failure warranting consideration for ECMO. Table 40.1 provides further details on the use of ECMO.

ECMO may be initiated for patients with primary cardiac or respiratory failure. The likelihood of meaningful recovery must be taken into account before initiation of ECMO because most patients who receive ECMO should have a reversible disease process with a reasonable chance of recovery. Therefore, it is recommended to consider use of ECMO, in the absence of contraindications, when the risk of mortality is estimated to be at least 50%. ECMO is indicated when the estimated risk of mortality exceeds 80%. Furthermore, before cannulation it is advisable to discuss with the family the duration for which ECMO will be continued (4,5).

The 2 primary modes for access when initiating ECMO are VV ECMO, which is used for isolated respiratory failure, and VA ECMO, which can provide

TABLE 40.1. Indications, Contraindications, and Common Complications of ECMO (VV or VA) in Critically Ill Adults

Potential Indications	Relative Contraindications[a]	Possible Complications
Failure to wean from cardiopulmonary bypass	Age >65 y	Stroke (hemorrhagic more common)
Cardiogenic shock	Mechanical ventilation for >7 d before cannulation	Hemorrhage (given use of heparin)
Before cardiac transplant	Nonrecoverable comorbidities (CNS hemorrhage, widespread malignancy, severe CNS damage)	Lower extremity ischemia (more common with VA ECMO)
Primary graft failure (cardiac or pulmonary)	Severe immunocompromise	Pneumothorax
Acute respiratory failure or ARDS		Pericardial tamponade Infection

Abbreviations: ARDS, acute respiratory distress syndrome; CNS, central nervous system; ECMO, extracorporeal membrane oxygenation; VA, venoarterial; VV, venovenous.
[a] *There are no absolute contraindications to extracorporeal membrane oxygenation.*

full cardiopulmonary support. Depending on the circuitry, ECMO can provide patients lifesaving oxygenation, carbon dioxide removal, and perfusion. In addition, the circuitry provides the possibility for inline ultrafiltration or continuous renal replacement therapy (or both).

Patients receiving ECMO therapy have an inherently higher risk of morbidity and death because ECMO initiation is usually considered for patients who need rescue after conventional treatment methods have failed and who have a high estimated mortality. Despite these considerations and the innate risks associated with receiving ECMO, survival rates greater than 50% have been reported for adults receiving ECMO for all causes, with up to 75% survival reported for patients receiving ECMO for H1N1 influenza in 2009.

REFERENCES

1. Combes A, Bacchetta M, Brodie D, Muller T, Pellegrino V. Extracorporeal membrane oxygenation for respiratory failure in adults. Curr Opin Crit Care. 2012 Feb;18(1):99-104.
2. Combes A, Brechot N, Luyt CE, Schmidt M. What is the niche for extracorporeal membrane oxygenation in severe acute respiratory distress syndrome? Curr Opin Crit Care. 2012 Oct;18(5):527-32.

Chest Pain and Respiratory Distress

DAVID W. BARBARA, MD,
AND WILLIAM J. MAUERMANN, MD

CASE PRESENTATION

An 83-year-old woman with a past medical history significant for hypertension and hyperlipidemia presented with a 1-day history of chest pain for which she did not seek medical attention. The following morning she awoke with respiratory distress, was taken to the emergency department, and was intubated for hypoxemic respiratory failure secondary to pulmonary edema. An electrocardiogram showed sinus tachycardia with prominent T waves in leads V_1 and V_2. A chest radiograph showed pulmonary infiltrates in the entire right lung and left lung base (Figure 41.1A). Cardiac catheterization showed only minimal coronary artery disease and severe mitral regurgitation. An intra-aortic balloon pump was placed. Transesophageal echocardiography showed a left ventricular ejection fraction of 70%, severe eccentric mitral regurgitation, a flail P2 scallop with torn chordae tendineae (Figure 41.1B), and systolic flow reversal noted in the right-sided, but not left-sided, pulmonary veins.

After a cardiac surgical consultation, the patient underwent an urgent operation for mitral valve repair. A P2 triangular resection and insertion of an annuloplasty band was performed, with only trivial residual mitral regurgitation (MR). Her postoperative course was prolonged because of pulmonary embolism, respiratory failure eventually requiring tracheostomy, and renal failure requiring dialysis, but she was ultimately discharged from the hospital on postoperative day 48.

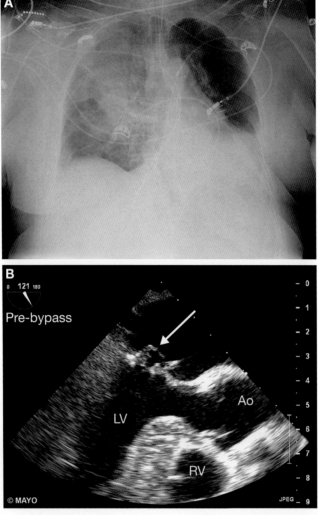

FIGURE 41.1. Acute Mitral Regurgitation. A, Chest radiograph shows pulmonary infiltrates in the entire right lung and left lung base. B, Transesophageal echocardiogram (midesophageal long-axis view) shows a flail P2 scallop (arrow) with torn chordae tendineae. Ao indicates aorta; LV, left ventricle; RV, right ventricle.

A follow-up transthoracic echocardiogram showed a left ventricular ejection fraction of 72% and trivial MR.

DISCUSSION

MR can be classified as acute or chronic. *Acute MR* involving native mitral valves has various causes that are either organic or functional (1). *Organic causes,* such as papillary muscle rupture, chordae tendineae rupture, or leaflet perforation, result in structural defects in the valve. Acute *functional MR* results from changes in the left ventricle and includes acute-onset cardiomyopathies with ventricular dilatation or ischemia involving the papillary muscle and its adjacent ventricular wall. Given the insufficient time for the left ventricle and left atrium to adapt to acute MR, patients typically present with hemodynamic instability and symptomatology directly related to the severity of MR. Therefore, treatment of severe acute MR is a medical and surgical emergency.

Specific causes of acute MR involving native mitral valves include myocardial ischemia, infective endocarditis, trauma, myxomatous disease, acute rheumatic fever, spontaneous or idiopathic chordae tendineae rupture, and acute nonischemic cardiomyopathy (eg, dilated cardiomyopathy, peripartum cardiomyopathy, and takotsubo cardiomyopathy) (1,2). In acute MR, a significant portion of the left ventricular stroke volume travels retrograde into the left atrium. There is no time for the left side of the heart to compensate by dilatation as is seen with chronic MR. Thus, patients present with depressed systemic output and severely increased left atrial pressure that results in pulmonary edema. The left ventricular ejection fraction may be hyperdynamic when MR is not associated with cardiomyopathy (ischemic or nonischemic), but systemic perfusion remains poor due to the MR. The clinical findings of severe acute MR are rapid onset of pulmonary edema and cardiogenic shock, including poor tissue perfusion and peripheral vasoconstriction. When patients have acute on chronic MR or less severe acute MR, symptomatology may not be as dramatic.

A systolic murmur and third heart sound are commonly heard, but up to 30% of patients with moderate or severe MR have been reported to have no audible murmur (3). This lack of auscultatory findings characteristic of MR is likely the result of a reduced pressure gradient between the left ventricle and the left atrium from systemic hypotension and acutely elevated left atrial pressure. Although electrocardiographic findings may indicate ischemia in patients with ischemic papillary muscle rupture, some patients do not have electrocardiographic abnormalities. The left atrial enlargement and atrial arrhythmias commonly seen with chronic MR are not typically present with acute MR. Chest radiography typically shows bilateral pulmonary edema with normal cardiac size; however, as observed in the patient described above, pulmonary edema may be unilateral in up to 25% of patients (4,5). Echocardiography helps to establish the diagnosis and mechanism of acute MR. When imaging with transthoracic echocardiography is inadequate, transesophageal echocardiography provides superior imaging. Although not indicated for all patients presenting with acute MR, cardiac catheterization is used 1) to define coronary artery anatomy and atherosclerosis (and to allow for potential intervention) when myocardial ischemia is considered a potential mechanism of MR and 2) to assess the need for concomitant coronary artery bypass surgery in patients with risk factors for coronary artery disease who are undergoing surgical repair of organic MR (1).

Medical treatment is directed at hemodynamic stabilization before operative treatment. Afterload reduction with a systemic vasodilator decreases the regurgitation fraction and increases the systemic cardiac output (1,2). Inotropic support may further improve cardiac output if ventricular function is depressed in the face of ischemia or cardiomyopathy. An intra-aortic balloon pump decreases afterload, thereby lessening the regurgitant fraction, and also improves coronary and systemic perfusion with balloon inflation in diastole. The intra-aortic balloon pump may be particularly useful in patients with acute MR from myocardial ischemia or cardiomyopathy (2). Although the majority of patients with severe acute MR may require operation, select patients with functional causes of MR may be amenable to medical treatment alone. For the majority of patients, early surgical intervention is recommended in the presence of hemodynamic compromise. When feasible, valvular repair is preferred over replacement (1,2).

REFERENCES

1. Stout KK, Verrier ED. Acute valvular regurgitation. Circulation. 2009 Jun 30;119(25):3232–41.

2. Mokadam NA, Stout KK, Verrier ED. Management of acute regurgitation in left-sided cardiac valves. Tex Heart Inst J. 2011;38(1):9–19.

3. Bursi F, Enriquez-Sarano M, Nkomo VT, Jacobsen SJ, Weston SA, Meverden RA, et al. Heart failure and death after myocardial infarction in the community: the emerging role of mitral regurgitation. Circulation. 2005 Jan 25;111(3):295–301. Epub 2005 Jan 17.

4. Warraich HJ, Bhatti UA, Shahul S, Pinto D, Liu D, Matyal R, et al. Unilateral pulmonary edema secondary to mitral valve perforation. Circulation. 2011 Nov 1;124(18):1994–5.

5. Attias D, Mansencal N, Auvert B, Vieillard-Baron A, Delos A, Lacombe P, et al. Prevalence, characteristics, and outcomes of patients presenting with cardiogenic unilateral pulmonary edema. Circulation. 2010 Sep 14;122(11):1109–15. Epub 2010 Aug 30.

Portal Venous Gas

BRENDAN T. WANTA, MD,
ARUN SUBRAMANIAN, MBBS,
AND MARK T. KEEGAN, MD

CASE PRESENTATION

A 70-year-old woman with recurrent high-grade ovarian cancer (for which she has undergone debulking surgery and chemotherapy), intermittent small-bowel obstruction, and atrial fibrillation was admitted to the hospital with nausea, vomiting, and diarrhea of several weeks' duration. She was transferred to the intensive care unit for treatment of rapidly developing respiratory failure that required intubation and ventilation and for treatment of distributive shock that required fluid and vasopressor therapy. Laboratory analyses showed a lactic acidosis and acidemia (lactate 5.9 mmol/L, pH 7.17, and bicarbonate 12 mmol/L), neutropenia, coagulopathy, and acute kidney injury. Emergent computed tomography of the abdomen showed pneumatosis intestinalis (PI) and portal venous gas (Figure 42.1). A diagnosis of presumed acute bowel ischemia was made, and the patient was appropriately resuscitated. Surgical options were discussed but not elected because of the patient's preadmission impaired functional status, poor prognosis, and family wishes. Comfort care was initiated, and the patient died shortly after. Autopsy findings included internal bowel herniation through thick adhesions and a large thrombus in the splenic vein.

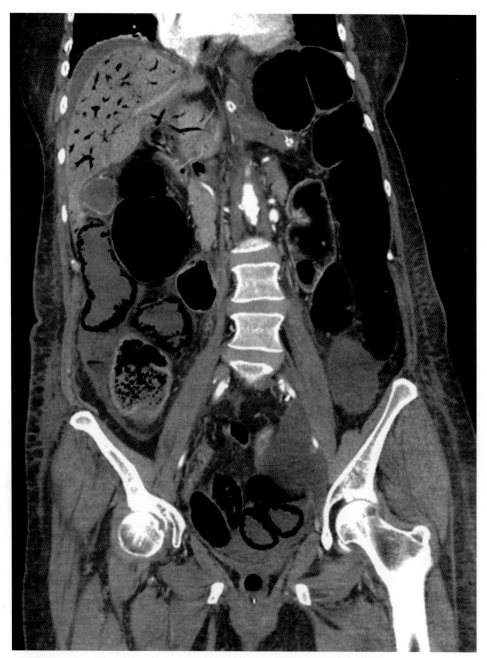

FIGURE 42.1. Pneumatosis Intestinalis. Computed tomography of the abdomen shows extensive pneumatosis involving multiple segments of the small bowel, mesenteric venous gas, and portal venous gas.

DISCUSSION

PI is the radiographic finding of air in the intestinal wall. It occurs in about 0.37% of patients who undergo radiographic imaging and is becoming a more common finding in critically ill patients (1). With the more frequent use of computed tomographic scanning, PI is increasingly reported (2).

BOX 42.1.
ETIOLOGY OF PNEUMATOSIS INTESTINALIS

Less worrisome

Gastrointestinal tract

   Peptic ulcer disease

   Inflammatory bowel disease

   Amyloidosis

Iatrogenic

   Endoscopy

   Surgery

   Sclerotherapy

Pharmacologic

   Immunotherapy

   Steroid therapy

   Chemotherapy

Pulmonary

   Asthma

   Chronic pulmonary disease

   Cystic fibrosis

More worrisome

Bowel necrosis

   Ischemia or infarction

   Sepsis

   Ingestion of caustic substance

Bowel obstruction

   Volvulus

   Pyloric stenosis

   Hirschsprung disease

Iatrogenic

   Stent perforation

Traumatic

   Blunt abdominal trauma

   Chest trauma

The spectrum of conditions that cause PI ranges from benign to life threatening. Intensivists need to distinguish between the conditions for which emergent surgical intervention is required and those in which the presence of PI is less clinically worrisome (Box 42.1).

The exact pathogenesis of PI has yet to be elucidated, but 2 major theories have been proposed. The first, a mechanical model, suggests that gas dissects through the bowel wall after a loss of mucosal integrity (eg, gastric ulcer), especially under conditions of increased intraluminal pressure (eg, in volvulus) (3). The second theory, a bacterial model, suggests that bacteria enter the submucosa through mucosal breaks and subsequently produce gas (4). In actuality, the pathogenesis is likely multifactorial. When PI is accompanied by visualization of portal venous gas, the likelihood of the presence of bowel necrosis greatly increases and may approach 90% because necrotic bowel provides a conduit for gas to enter the portal venous system (3-5). In this situation, prompt surgical management is usually the treatment of choice.

REFERENCES

1. Morris MS, Gee AC, Cho SD, Limbaugh K, Underwood S, Ham B, et al. Management and outcome of pneumatosis intestinalis. Am J Surg. 2008 May;195(5):679–82.

2. Pieterse AS, Leong AS, Rowland R. The mucosal changes and pathogenesis of pneumatosis cystoides intestinalis. Hum Pathol. 1985 Jul;16(7):683–8.

3. Yale CE. Etiology of pneumatosis cystoides intestinalis. Surg Clin North Am. 1975 Dec;55(6):1297–302.

4. Pear BL. Pneumatosis intestinalis: a review. Radiology. 1998 Apr;207(1):13–9.

5. Wiesner W, Mortele KJ, Glickman JN, Ji H, Ros PR. Pneumatosis intestinalis and portomesenteric venous gas in intestinal ischemia: correlation of CT findings with severity of ischemia and clinical outcome. AJR Am J Roentgenol. 2001 Dec;177(6):1319–23.

Acute Respiratory Failure in a Stem Cell Transplant Patient

CHANNING C. TWYNER, MD, AND ARUN SUBRAMANIAN, MBBS

CASE PRESENTATION

A 59-year-old man presented with neutropenic fever, fatigue, rash, and marked diarrhea 9 days after undergoing autologous stem cell transplant (ASCT) for multiple myeloma. At admission, he was profoundly neutropenic (leukocyte count 0.1×10^9/L). A workup for infection was instituted, and therapy was begun with broad-spectrum antimicrobials and intravenous fluid repletion. Blood, sputum, and urine culture results were negative. Chest radiography did not show any infiltrate. Over the next 4 days, although his leukocyte count increased to 1.3×10^9/L, his clinical status deteriorated. He had worsening dyspnea, hypoxia, and oliguria, necessitating transfer to the intensive care unit (ICU). Portable chest radiography showed new bilateral interstitial infiltrates (Figure 43.1). After other differential diagnoses were carefully considered, an empirical diagnosis of periengraftment respiratory distress syndrome (PERDS) was made, and high doses of daily corticosteroids were begun. Rapid clinical and radiographic improvement occurred over the next week, and the patient was discharged with an oral corticosteroid taper.

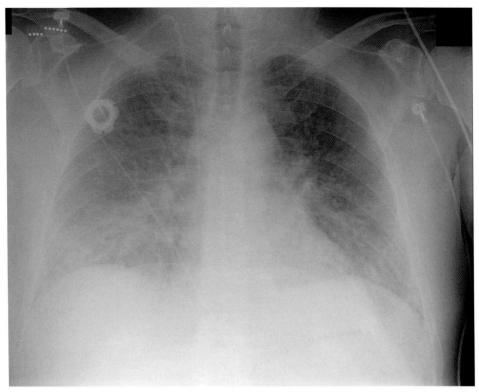

FIGURE 43.1. Portable Chest Radiograph. The patient presented with acute dyspnea and hypoxia 13 days after undergoing autologous stem cell transplant.

DISCUSSION

After conditioning chemotherapy and ASCT, hematopoietic stem cells begin to form neutrophils, as evidenced by their appearance in the peripheral blood. This period of myeloid restitution is *neutrophil engraftment*, defined as an absolute neutrophil count greater than 0.5×10^9/L on 3 or more consecutive days after ASCT. It is postulated that during this phase, a "cytokine storm" may drive a constellation of symptoms, including noninfectious fever, skin rash, diarrhea, and increased capillary permeability (1). This "engraftment syndrome" is associated with an increased risk of respiratory failure, with or without multisystem organ failure. If lung injury develops within 4 to 25 days after transplant (median, 11 days), in the absence of infectious and cardiac causes, the diagnosis of PERDS is suggested and corticosteroid therapy is indicated (2).

The approach to acute pulmonary edema should start with a history and physical examination focused on noncardiogenic and cardiogenic causes of pulmonary edema. Congestive heart failure, acute myocardial infarction, heart valve disease, and volume overload are causes of cardiogenic pulmonary edema. Cardiogenic causes are ruled out with an unremarkable electrocardiogram and transthoracic echocardiogram as well as normal levels of cardiac troponins and brain natriuretic peptide (3). After cardiogenic causes have been ruled out, noncardiogenic causes due to capillary leak should be considered. The differential diagnosis for noncardiogenic pulmonary edema is broad and highlights the importance of the history and physical examination.

A multitude of pulmonary complications can occur in stem cell transplant patients, so it is important to recognize the complications that respond rapidly to treatment. The patient described above illustrates that PERDS can be easily overlooked unless it is deliberately considered in a patient with fever, rash, hypoxia, and capillary leak soon after neutrophil engraftment. Timely corticosteroid therapy can help patients avoid the need for mechanical ventilation, multiple tests, or a prolonged ICU stay and facilitate a dramatically favorable outcome compared to other morbid complications of bone marrow transplant. The diagnostic criteria are not uniform, so the reported incidence in various series ranges from 7% to 59% (4). The similarity of the clinical presentation and the absence of diagnostic tests can pose a challenge in distinguishing PERDS from more frequently encountered sequelae in stem cell transplant patients. Infectious and noninfectious causes must be excluded (eg, transfusion-related acute lung injury, transfusion-associated circulatory overload, cardiogenic pulmonary edema, diffuse alveolar hemorrhage, and idiopathic pneumonia syndrome) (5).

REFERENCES

1. Capizzi SA, Kumar S, Huneke NE, Gertz MA, Inwards DJ, Litzow MR, et al. Peri-engraftment respiratory distress syndrome during autologous hematopoietic stem cell transplantation. Bone Marrow Transplant. 2001 Jun;27(12):1299–303.

2. Afessa B, Peters SG. Noninfectious pneumonitis after blood and marrow transplant. Curr Opin Oncol. 2008 Mar;20(2):227–33.

3. Ware LB, Matthay MA. Clinical practice: acute pulmonary edema. N Engl J Med. 2005 Dec 29;353(26):2788–96.

4. Carreras E, Fernandez-Aviles F, Silva L, Guerrero M, Fernandez de Larrea C, Martinez C, et al. Engraftment syndrome after auto-SCT: analysis of diagnostic criteria and risk factors in a large series from a single center. Bone Marrow Transplant. 2010 Sep;45(9):1417–22. Epub 2010 Jan 11.

5. Afessa B, Peters SG. Major complications following hematopoietic stem cell transplantation. Semin Respir Crit Care Med. 2006 Jun;27(3):297–309.

Flail Chest

SUMEDH S. HOSKOTE, MBBS, JOHN C. O'HORO, MD, MPH, AND CRAIG E. DANIELS, MD

CASE PRESENTATION

A 60-year-old woman was admitted to the coronary care unit after return of spontaneous circulation with successful cardiopulmonary resuscitation (CPR) for out-of-hospital pulseless electrical activity cardiac arrest at a skilled nursing facility. Duration of CPR was approximately 30 minutes. The patient had a history of breast cancer (she had undergone bilateral mastectomies and chemotherapy), renal transplant for autosomal dominant polycystic kidney disease, and hypertension. After admission and attempted hemodynamic stabilization, she was treated for 24 hours with therapeutic hypothermia, which included fentanyl and midazolam sedation. She was found to have anuric acute kidney injury and septic shock, so she was given vasopressors, antibiotics, and continuous renal replacement therapy.

On day 3, the patient slowly regained consciousness but was noted to be tachypneic and dyssynchronous with mechanical ventilation. Arterial blood gas results showed mixed respiratory and metabolic acidosis. On physical examination, she was drowsy but able to follow some simple commands. Cardiac auscultation was normal. Chest examination was notable for bilateral rhonchi. With mechanical ventilation and spontaneous breathing (continuous positive airway pressure 5 cm H_2O, with pressure support ventilation 5 cm H_2O), the sternal segment of the anterior thoracic chest wall was observed to move paradoxically inward during inspiration. Abdominal examination findings were normal. Computed tomography of the chest confirmed the clinical diagnosis of flail chest, with bilateral rib fractures involving ribs 2 through 9. The patient had bibasilar effusions with overlying infiltrate likely secondary to aspiration pneumonitis, and pulmonary contusion was not noted. The flail chest resulted in failure of spontaneous breathing trials despite adequate analgesia. A prolonged strategy to liberate the patient from mechanical ventilation included increased positive end-expiratory pressure (PEEP) and analgesia. The patient's neurologic outcome, however, was not favorable and further aggressive measures, such as epidural block or surgical rib fixation, were not pursued. The patient's family elected for transitioning to comfort measures, and the patient died.

DISCUSSION

Flail chest refers to a deformity of the chest wall caused by fracture of at least 3 consecutive ribs, each broken at 2 or more places. Flail chest may cause or exacerbate respiratory failure through paradoxical chest wall motion during the phases of respiration: The characteristic physical examination finding is that the flail segment moves inward during inspiration and outward during expiration. Management of flail chest requires attention to clinical recognition, mechanical ventilation, analgesia, and, in certain circumstances, surgical fixation.

Flail chest injuries occur most often with trauma. However, as the population of cardiac arrest survivors increases, post-CPR flail chest is being observed more frequently. The extent of injury after CPR can be unilateral or bilateral, or it may involve the sternum as in the patient described above. Flail segments produce a severe restrictive ventilatory defect that leads to ineffective ventilation, with resultant hypoventilation and hypercarbia. Diagnosis is especially challenging when patients have undergone CPR because they are frequently comatose or sedated and unable to report pain or tenderness over the fractured ribs. In practice, physical examination findings may be the only clues to the diagnosis because rib fractures are routinely missed with chest radiography (1). Paradoxical chest wall motion is the characteristic examination finding in patients who have flail chest; further support for the diagnosis is provided by finding external signs of trauma, including crepitus and palpable deformities. Bedside pulmonary function assessments are useful in assessing the risk of respiratory failure; these include inspiratory and expiratory forces and vital capacity.

Analgesia is the cornerstone of flail chest management. Intravenous opiates are often used and are administered with intermittent boluses, infusions, or patient-controlled analgesia pumps. However, recent practice has moved away from using opiates alone because of their many adverse effects at high doses. Placement of an epidural catheter for continuous infusion of local anesthetic with or without opiates has been shown to be superior to intravenous opiates and is currently the standard of care in treating pain associated with flail chest (2). Intercostal nerve blocks with local anesthetics may also be used for smaller flail segments.

Pulmonary contusion occurs in about 30% to 75% of all blunt thoracic traumas and is a major cause of morbidity and mortality among patients with thoracic trauma and flail chest (3,4). Thus, pulmonary contusion must be ruled out in every patient with flail chest, and these 2 conditions should essentially be managed as 1. The Eastern Association for the Surgery of Trauma recommends that patients with flail chest and underlying pulmonary contusion should not undergo excessive fluid restriction but should be resuscitated as necessary with isotonic crystalloid or colloid solution to maintain signs of adequate tissue perfusion (4). After a patient is adequately resuscitated, unnecessary fluid administration should be meticulously avoided (4). There is no recommendation for the use of corticosteroids in the treatment of flail chest or pulmonary contusion (4). Patients with respiratory failure should be supported with mechanical ventilation (noninvasive or invasive) to provide PEEP (3,4). The provision of modest levels of PEEP, in addition to increasing functional residual capacity and improving oxygenation, maintains the lung partially inflated in expiration, thus splinting the collapsing flail segment. This strategy, *internal stabilization*, is in contrast to external (surgical) fixation or stabilization of the thoracic cage. Bronchial hygiene to facilitate secretion clearance and prevent mucous plugging is also important in management. A multidisciplinary team approach for the treatment of chest wall injuries may improve outcome and should be considered where feasible (4).

Surgical rib fixation is controversial and not universally used for treating flail chest. A recent meta-analysis showed that patients who received surgical fixation as the initial treatment had decreased mortality, length of stay, duration of mechanical ventilation, need for tracheostomy, and incidence of pneumonia (5). Surgical fixation may be considered for patients with flail chest who continue to have poor pulmonary function despite conservative management.

The mechanical injury of flail chest may also be associated with hemothorax or pneumothorax, which is managed with chest tube insertion. For patients who have flail chest and are being treated with mechanical ventilation, the value of prophylactic chest tube insertion is not certain.

REFERENCES

1. Lederer W, Mair D, Rabl W, Baubin M. Frequency of rib and sternum fractures associated with out-of-hospital cardiopulmonary resuscitation is underestimated by conventional chest X-ray. Resuscitation. 2004 Feb;60(2):157–62.

2. Bulger EM, Edwards T, Klotz P, Jurkovich GJ. Epidural analgesia improves outcome after multiple rib fractures. Surgery. 2004 Aug;136(2):426–30.

3. Dehghan N, de Mestral C, McKee MD, Schemitsch EH, Nathens A. Flail chest injuries: a review of outcomes and treatment practices from the National Trauma Data Bank. J Trauma Acute Care Surg. 2014 Feb;76(2):462–8.

4. Simon B, Ebert J, Bokhari F, Capella J, Emhoff T, Hayward T 3rd, et al; Eastern Association for the Surgery of Trauma. Management of pulmonary contusion and flail chest: an Eastern Association for the Surgery of Trauma practice management guideline. J Trauma Acute Care Surg. 2012 Nov;73(5 Suppl 4):S351–61.

5. Leinicke JA, Elmore L, Freeman BD, Colditz GA. Operative management of rib fractures in the setting of flail chest: a systematic review and meta-analysis. Ann Surg. 2013 Dec;258(6):914–21.

Coma

MUHAMMAD A. RISHI, MBBS,
SARAH J. LEE, MD, MPH,
AND TENG MOUA, MD

CASE PRESENTATION

A 68-year-old man with a past medical history of a fall, which resulted in a complex acetabular-pelvic fracture 3 weeks earlier, presented to the emergency department after being found hypotensive in a nursing home.

At his previous admission, the patient had undergone pericardiocentesis, for a benign chronic pericardial effusion of unknown cause, and traction pin placement for the complex acetabular-pelvic fracture. In the emergency department, during the current admission, he was found to have worsening anemia with hypotension, a hemoglobin level of 6.4 g/dL, a serum sodium level of 134 mmol/L, and an enlarging subcutaneous and intrapelvic hematoma. His current medications included metoprolol, oxycodone, and prophylactic enoxaparin.

The patient was resuscitated with red blood cells, fresh frozen plasma, and fluids, with subsequent hemodynamic stabilization. He was then transferred for pelvic angiography, which showed no active extravasation of contrast medium. He was subsequently transferred to the intensive care unit (ICU) for further management.

Progressive lethargy and somnolence developed over the course of the hospitalization, and the patient became difficult to arouse on day 5 of his ICU stay. He was found to have delayed deep tendon reflexes. The rest of the examination findings were unremarkable. The differential diagnosis for somnolence in a hospitalized patient is broad and includes cardiovascular, structural, infectious, and toxic-metabolic causes. A computerized tomographic scan of the head did not show any acute intracranial pathologic features. As part of the workup for profound somnolence, a serum thyrotropin level was ordered; the result was 369.1 mIU/L (reference range, 0.5-4.4 mIU/L). The diagnosis was myxedema coma, likely precipitated by acute hemorrhagic shock. When the patient was given thyroid replacement therapy (a combination of intravenous triiodothyronine [T$_3$] and thyroxine [T$_4$]), his symptoms improved dramatically. Subsequent inquiry elicited a remote past history of untreated hypothyroidism.

DISCUSSION

Myxedema coma is a rare manifestation of extreme hypothyroidism. The reported incidence is 0.22 per million per year (1). It is seen most commonly in hospitalized elderly female patients who have a history of hypothyroidism. Myxedema coma is a life-threatening condition (1), and improving survival of patients with myxedema coma depends on understanding its pathogenesis and recognizing its clinical presentation, with early and accurate diagnosis and intervention.

The typical presentation of patients with myxedema coma is an acute systemic illness superimposed on previously undiagnosed or untreated hypothyroidism (2). The 2 pathognomonic features of myxedema coma are hypothermia (often profound, to 26°C) and loss of consciousness. Patients may be afebrile or hypothermic despite underlying severe infection.

Although coma is the classic clinical presentation, paranoia, hallucinations (myxedema madness), disorientation, or depression have also been described. Neurologic findings may also include cerebellar signs and poor memory and recall, or possibly amnesia, with electroencephalography showing low-amplitude, reduced alpha-wave activity due to the reduced metabolic activity of the brain.

Hypoventilation is caused by the combined effect of a reduced hypoxic respiratory drive and a depressed ventilatory response to hypercapnia. Pleural effusions or ascites may also contribute to reduced minute ventilation. After they are intubated, patients often need prolonged mechanical ventilation. They also have an increased risk of cardiogenic shock and arrhythmias. Pericardial effusions, which are often occult and rich in mucopolysaccharides, have been described. The pericardial effusion in the patient described above was likely related to his severe hypothyroidism. Commonly described electrocardiographic findings include low voltage, bradycardia, flattened or inverted T waves, various degrees of heart block, and an increased QT interval.

Hyponatremia is often reported and results from increased serum levels of antidiuretic hormone and impaired water diuresis. Gastric atony, impaired peristalsis, and paralytic ileus have also been described and are thought to result from infiltration of the gastrointestinal wall by mucopolysaccharides and from muscularis edema.

Acquired von Willebrand disease (type 1) and reduced synthesis of factors V, VII, VIII, IX, and X increase the risk of bleeding in patients with severe hypothyroidism. Patients also have an increased preponderance for severe infections, including septic shock, which is thought to result from neutropenia and a reduced cell-mediated response. An increased concentration of serum thyrotropin is the most important laboratory evidence for the diagnosis. However, the presence of severe systemic illness or treatment with drugs such as vasopressors or corticosteroids may decrease the thyrotropin levels, making interpretation of the test results difficult.

Myxedema coma is a medical emergency that requires a multipronged approach to management in an ICU (3). Respiratory failure is common, so that airway management is of paramount importance. Hypotension often improves with thyroid replacement therapy, but patients may initially require volume resuscitation. Hypothermia is treated with passive rewarming, and hyponatremia may need careful correction with saline solution. Associated problems, including infection, congestive heart failure, diabetes mellitus, or hypertension, also require treatment.

Adequate data from clinical studies are not available, and controlled trials would be difficult to perform, so the optimal thyroid replacement strategy is unknown. When T_4 is administered alone, the plasma level fluctuates less, but it also has a slower onset of action than T_3. A relatively conservative and rational approach is to provide both T_4 and T_3 as combination therapy. A bolus of 4 mg/kg lean body weight (or 200-300 mg) of intravenous T_4 is administered, followed by 100 mg given after 24 hours. By day 3, the dose is reduced to a daily maintenance dose of 50 mg. The oral route can be used as soon as the patient is able. When the initial dose of T_4 is administered, a bolus of 10 mg of T_3 is given intravenously and continued at 10 mg every 8 to 12 hours until the patient is conscious and taking maintenance T_4. Subsequently, T_3 therapy can be stopped.

Patients with myxedema coma have a poor prognosis (4), but with advances in critical care, mortality has been decreased to 20% to 25% from a previous high of 60% to 70%. Severe hypothermia and hypotension are poor prognostic indicators.

REFERENCES

1. Rodriguez I, Fluiters E, Perez-Mendez LF, Luna R, Paramo C, Garcia-Mayor RV. Factors associated with mortality of patients with myxoedema coma: prospective study in 11 cases treated in a single institution. J Endocrinol. 2004 Feb;180(2):347–50.
2. Kwaku MP, Burman KD. Myxedema coma. J Intensive Care Med. 2007 Jul-Aug;22(4):224–31.
3. Reinhardt W, Mann K. [Incidence, clinical picture and treatment of hypothyroid coma: results of a survey]. Med Klin (Munich). 1997 Sep 15;92(9):521–4. German.
4. Yamamoto T, Fukuyama J, Fujiyoshi A. Factors associated with mortality of myxedema coma: report of eight cases and literature survey. Thyroid. 1999 Dec;9(12):1167–74.

A Bleeding Disorder

JOHN C. O'HORO, MD, MPH, AND PHILIPPE R. BAUER, MD, PhD

CASE PRESENTATION

An 81-year-old man who had a diagnosis of coronary artery disease and was receiving dual antiplatelet therapy presented to his local primary care provider for discolorations and bruises in his fingers and toes. Initial findings were negative aside from hematuria and an elevated D-dimer level that led to computed tomographic angiography for pulmonary embolism and to ultrasonography for deep vein thrombosis; results of both imaging studies were negative. His aspirin and clopidogrel therapy was stopped, and he was observed as an outpatient. However, he continued to feel malaise, his hematuria worsened, and his urinalysis results were concerning for infection. He was admitted for treatment of presumed urosepsis.

After admission, blood cultures grew *Staphylococcus* species, and he was given appropriate antibiotics. He was dismissed to a skilled nursing facility, where he had continued difficulty with bleeding from his venipuncture sites and worsening hematuria. Subsequently, he was transferred to a tertiary care center for evaluation and management of presumed disseminated intravascular coagulation (DIC).

On arrival, he was anemic (hemoglobin 6.8 g/dL), and his platelet count (244×10^9/L) was within the reference range. On physical examination, he had large areas of ecchymoses over his chest, abdomen, arms, and legs. Results of the initial coagulation studies were D-dimer level greater than 2,000 ng/mL, fibrino-gen 533 mg/dL, international normalized ratio 1.0, and activated partial throm-boplastin time (aPTT) 68 seconds. The patient received a transfusion and was treated empirically with fresh frozen plasma and desmopressin acetate for ongo-ing bleeding. His status stabilized, a hematologist was consulted, and further coagulation tests were performed.

A mixing study incompletely corrected the aPTT to 47 seconds. The dilute Russell viper venom time (dRVVT) was normal. Examination of factor activities showed a decrease in factor VIII activity to less than 1%. Activity for factors IX, XI, and XII was normal. The patient was found to have a factor VIII inhibitor and was treated with corticosteroids, cyclophosphamide, and activated prothrombin complex concentrates. His bleeding status stabilized, and he was discharged the next week with close follow-up with a hematologist.

DISCUSSION

Abnormal coagulation study findings can result from several critical illnesses. The broad differential diagnosis of these disorders requires a thorough history, physi-cal examination, and further laboratory investigations appropriate for the patient's clinical presentation.

In treating a critically ill patient who has a coagulopathy, the first step is to control all major sources of bleeding. Physical examination to identify areas of blood loss, such as hemoperitoneum, thigh hematoma, gastrointestinal tract blood loss, or massive hemoptysis, should be followed by attempting hemostasis with an appropriate procedural intervention, such as direct pressure, endoscopy, or surgery. The use of blood products should be guided by the patient's clinical course and appearance rather than solely correction of laboratory values. When hemostasis is achieved, the reason for coagulopathy must be determined to allow for effective treatment.

Identifying the type of defect requires an understanding of the clotting process (Figure 46.1). Both an adequate number of functional platelets and operational coagulation pathways are essential for creating and maintaining a stable clot. Physical examination findings can provide clues to the type of disorder; mucocu-taneous bleeding and petechiae are typical of platelet disorders, while coagulation cascade defects more typically create large, spreading deep tissue ecchymoses and hematomas.

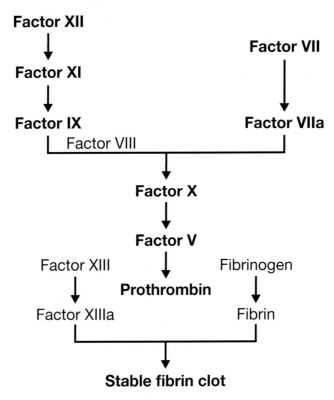

FIGURE 46.1. Coagulation Process. The intrinsic pathway, starting with factor XII, is assessed by the activated partial thromboplastin time. The extrinsic pathway, starting with activation of factor VII (to factor VIIa), is more closely associated with the prothrombin time. Both are affected by the common pathway, from factor X through formation of a clot. Administration of recombinant factor VIIa or activated prothrombin complexes bypasses the intrinsic pathway, which is rendered nonfunctional by a factor VIII inhibitor, and allows for "rescue" of the clotting cascade.

A platelet count is an essential first laboratory test to exclude thrombocytopenia. Functional platelet tests, such as bleeding time and platelet function analyzers, are not commonly used or recommended unless there are specific concerns with platelet function. Prothrombin time (PT) and aPTT provide insights into the functioning of the intrinsic and extrinsic coagulation cascades. If a defect in the coagulation cascade is suspected, possible causes are deficiencies or inhibitors. Mixing studies are used to investigate for inhibitors by combining normal and patient plasma, testing PT and aPTT, and seeing whether the times normalize. If the problem is a deficiency, the times will normalize, whereas if an inhibitor is involved, the times will not normalize or will only partially normalize. A unique case is the factor VIII inhibitors, which correct the aPTT immediately, but then the aPPT is prolonged after 60 to 120 minutes of incubation. This led to the creation of the Bethesda assay, in which serial dilutions of patient plasma are mixed with normal plasma and incubated for 2 hours at 37°C; factor VIII activity is then assessed, and the reciprocal dilution of plasma with 50% factor VII activity is reported (1).

If aPTT alone is prolonged, lupus anticoagulant is tested with the dRVVT, although the clinical appearance of patients with lupus anticoagulant is thrombosis rather than bleeding. If bleeding is present, the clinical presentation is more consistent with acquired hemophilia; other specific factor inhibitors can then be tested as well, with factor VIII being the most common.

Thromboelastography, fibrinogen, and D-dimer testing are used to examine for active fibrinolysis, as occurs in DIC. These additional tests should be ordered as clinically appropriate for a more extensive workup for DIC.

The most common acquired inhibitors interfere with factor VIII activity in acquired hemophilia, which occurs in 1 per 1 million people annually (1,2). The reason for autoantibody production against this factor is unknown, but the majority of patients are either 1) older than 50 years or 2) younger and pregnant or postpartum. There is a positive correlation with other autoimmune diseases, but in half the patients, no such disease is present (2,3).

Treatment of factor VIII inhibitor involves both achieving hemostasis and eliminating the inhibitor. Initial treatment requires bypassing factor VIII with activated prothrombin complex concentrates, factor VIII concentrates, or desmopressin. When hemostasis is achieved, cyclophosphamide can be used in combination with corticosteroids as an immunosuppressant to remove the inhibitor (1).

REFERENCES

1. Delgado J, Jimenez-Yuste V, Hernandez-Navarro F, Villar A. Acquired haemophilia: review and meta-analysis focused on therapy and prognostic factors. Br J Haematol. 2003 Apr;121(1):21–35.

2. Collins P, Macartney N, Davies R, Lees S, Giddings J, Majer R. A population based, unselected, consecutive cohort of patients with acquired haemophilia A. Br J Haematol. 2004 Jan;124(1):86–90.

3. Collins PW, Hirsch S, Baglin TP, Dolan G, Hanley J, Makris M, et al; UK Haemophilia Centre Doctors' Organisation. Acquired hemophilia A in the United Kingdom: a 2-year national surveillance study by the United Kingdom Haemophilia Centre Doctors' Organisation. Blood. 2007 Mar 1;109(5):1870–7. Epub 2006 Oct 17.

A Cardiopulmonary
Resuscitation Complication

JOHN C. O'HORO, MD, MPH,
SUMEDH S. HOSKOTE, MBBS,
AND HIROSHI SEKIGUCHI, MD

CASE PRESENTATION

A 94-year-old woman with coronary artery disease and bladder cancer became light-headed 10 minutes after receiving an intravenous contrast agent for a computed tomographic (CT) urogram. Subsequently, she became unresponsive and pulseless. She underwent 5 minutes of cardiopulmonary resuscitation (CPR), during which no shock was advised by an automatic external defibrillator. She was taken to the emergency department after return of spontaneous circulation (ROSC) was achieved. Chest radiography showed interstitial infiltrates bilaterally without evidence of pneumothorax. CT angiography of the chest was negative for pulmonary embolism; however, it showed a small left apical pneumothorax, acute fractures bilaterally of ribs 3 through 6, and interlobular septal thickening with diffuse ground-glass opacities suggestive of pulmonary edema. Results from electrocardiography and laboratory testing were unremarkable except for frequent premature ventricular complexes and an elevated level of troponin. The patient became progressively dyspneic and was transferred to the intensive care unit.

In the intensive care unit, chest radiography showed worsening bilateral pulmonary infiltrates but no apparent pneumothorax. Laboratory testing showed marked leukocytosis and a normal lactate level. The patient became progressively hypoxemic and hypotensive and was given noninvasive positive pressure ventilation (PPV) and vasopressors. Subsequently, she was intubated for worsening hypoxemic and hypercapnic respiratory failure. Immediately after intubation, she had a pulseless electrical activity (PEA) arrest. Although ROSC was achieved after a few cycles of CPR, the patient had another PEA arrest. Emergent needle thoracostomy was performed in the left anterior thorax, which resulted in an immediate ROSC and confirmed the diagnosis of tension pneumothorax. A chest tube was placed for further chest decompression.

DISCUSSION

This patient sustained bilateral rib fractures and occult pneumothorax secondary to CPR, which is an underrecognized cause of blunt cardiopulmonary injuries. Rib fracture is seen in approximately 30% of patients (1). Other thoracic and pulmonary injuries include pulmonary bone marrow or fat emboli (in 19% of patients), sternum fracture (in 15%), aspiration (in 11%), and mediastinal bleeding (in 10%) (1). Common cardiovascular injuries include coronary artery rupture or laceration and pericardial injuries (1). In an autopsy series (1), an evident pneumothorax was seen in 3% of nonsurvivors, but the actual pneumothorax rate is likely higher.

Occult pneumothorax, defined as pneumothorax seen on CT but not suspected on chest radiography, can be missed at autopsy if it is very small, and it may not be diagnosed in patients who cannot undergo a CT scan after CPR. In fact, occult pneumothorax has been increasingly detected because of the nearly routine use of CT with trauma patients (2). As in the patient described above, an occult pneumothorax can become a tension pneumothorax with PPV. However, a randomized study on blunt trauma populations (2) suggested that occult pneumothorax in patients undergoing PPV may be safely observed without the need for urgent pleural drainage.

The conventional view is that tension pneumothorax leads to a rapid increase in intrapleural pressure, which causes mechanical physiologic changes that are seen almost exclusively in patients undergoing PPV (3). In nonassisted, spontaneously breathing patients, intrapleural pressure cannot exceed atmospheric pressure during inspiration; hence, pneumothorax results in progressive respiratory failure and hypoxemia but not in sudden cardiovascular collapse (3).

Tension pneumothorax is a clinical diagnosis that is confirmed only with a reversal of respiratory and hemodynamic compromise on thoracic decompression (3). Nonetheless, a thorough, useful clinical examination should include vital signs, auscultation for diminished or absent breath sounds, and bedside ultrasonography to assess the lung sliding. However, if the diagnosis is suspected and the patient is hemodynamically unstable, empirical treatment should not be delayed.

Initial treatment of tension pneumothorax is thoracic decompression with a needle thoracostomy. It has been recommended to insert a 14- or 16-gauge angiocatheter into the second intercostal space (ICS) along the midclavicular line. However, the reported failure rate of needle thoracostomy is relatively high because of inadequate catheter length to reach the pleural cavity, catheter kinking, occlusion, and dislodgment (4). Studies have suggested that a longer needle may be required for insertion at the second ICS in up to 40% of patients and that the fifth ICS at the anterior axillary line may be more accessible and carry a higher success rate (4). Consequently, an urgent tube thoracostomy may be necessary when the level of suspicion is high if a needle thoracostomy does not reverse the hemodynamic compromise.

In general, a tube thoracostomy is recommended after a needle thoracostomy in hemodynamically unstable patients. A tube thoracostomy allows effective treatment of unresolved pneumothorax; averts recurrent tension pneumothorax due to angiocatheter kinking, occlusion, or dislodgment; and prevents tension hemopneumothorax in the presence of concurrent intrathoracic bleeding. In recent studies, not all trauma patients who underwent a needle thoracostomy required a tube thoracotomy when they were hemodynamically stable (2).

In summary, tension pneumothorax can cause a PEA arrest in patients who have undergone CPR for an initial cardiopulmonary arrest. Tension pneumothorax is a life-threatening obstructive shock that requires early recognition and immediate thoracic decompression. Clinicians should be aware of the benefits and limitations of a needle thoracostomy in addition to the indication for a tube thoracostomy.

REFERENCES

1. Miller AC, Rosati SF, Suffredini AF, Schrump DS. A systematic review and pooled analysis of CPR-associated cardiovascular and thoracic injuries. Resuscitation. 2014 Jun;85(6):724–31. Epub 2014 Feb 10.

2. Kirkpatrick AW, Rizoli S, Ouellet JF, Roberts DJ, Sirois M, Ball CG, et al; Canadian Trauma Trials Collaborative and the Research Committee of the Trauma Association of Canada. Occult pneumothoraces in critical care: a prospective multicenter randomized controlled trial of pleural drainage for mechanically ventilated trauma patients with occult pneumothoraces. J Trauma Acute Care Surg. 2013 Mar;74(3):747–54.

3. Leigh-Smith S, Harris T. Tension pneumothorax: time for a re-think? Emerg Med J. 2005 Jan;22(1):8–16.

4. Inaba K, Ives C, McClure K, Branco BC, Eckstein M, Shatz D, et al. Radiologic evaluation of alternative sites for needle decompression of tension pneumothorax. Arch Surg. 2012 Sep;147(9):813–8.

Severe Influenza A–Associated Acute Respiratory Distress Syndrome

RUDY M. TEDJA, DO, AND CRAIG E. DANIELS, MD

CASE PRESENTATION

A 36-year-old man with a history of Hodgkin lymphoma 11 years ago was transferred to the intensive care unit (ICU) at a tertiary care center for management of acute respiratory distress syndrome (ARDS) caused by influenza A virus. ARDS was diagnosed 5 days before the transfer. The patient was found to have methicillin-resistant *Staphylococcus aureus* growth with elevated levels of eosinophils (72%) in the bronchoalveolar fluid. Computed tomography of the chest showed bilateral pneumonitis with peripheral infiltrates. The patient was treated with oseltamivir, vancomycin, and piperacillin-tazobactam. Echocardiography showed normal cardiac function. Upon arrival in the ICU, the patient was intubated and sedated. Ventilator settings were volume-cycled, assist-control, low tidal volume ventilation (6 mL/kg predicted body weight) with fraction of inspired oxygen (FIO_2) of 100% and positive end-expiratory pressure (PEEP) of 15 cm H_2O. The Pao_2/FIO_2 ratio was 68 mm Hg. The patient was subsequently paralyzed with an infusion of cisatracurium, a neuromuscular blocker (NMB), and given alprostadil as an inhaled vasodilator to improve oxygenation. Extracorporeal membrane oxygenation (ECMO) was considered but was deferred in favor of conventional ARDS management. On hospital day 2, the patient remained profoundly hypoxemic despite several attempted ventilatory strategies. Prone ventilation was initiated.

On hospital day 5, the patient was making good clinical progress. FIO_2 had improved to 50%, and PEEP was 10 cm H_2O. Chest radiography showed improvement of the bilateral lung infiltrates. The patient was weaned from both prone ventilation and inhaled vasodilatory therapies. However, because of his restrictive lung physiology, high dead space, and work of breathing, the patient could not be weaned from the mechanical ventilator. A percutaneous tracheostomy was placed. His ICU course was further complicated with ventilator-associated events, highly persistent fever, pancytopenia, rash, and ICU delirium. An exhaustive evaluation of fever, including bone marrow and skin biopsies, was performed but did not lead to a certain diagnosis. The patient tested persistently positive for influenza A virus by polymerase chain reaction on bronchoalveolar fluid; high-dose oseltamivir (150 mg oral twice daily) was continued. On hospital day 14, the patient remained critically ill, and his condition continued to deteriorate. Prone ventilation was resumed with the goal of improving his oxygenation. ECMO was again considered but was deferred after consideration of multiple medical and preference factors. The family eventually withdrew care and the patient died.

DISCUSSION

ARDS is a life-threatening respiratory condition characterized by diffuse inflammatory lung injury leading to profound hypoxemia and stiff lungs. It occurs typically within 6 to 72 hours after an inciting event. Influenza A viral pneumonia can progress to severe ARDS with multisystem organ failure, as seen during the 2009-2010 pandemic with H1N1 influenza A virus. Extensive studies on therapeutic modalities have found no effective pharmacologic therapies. Supportive care with mechanical ventilation remains the cornerstone of treatment.

Low tidal volume ventilation is the only strategy that has been shown to improve mortality (1). Along with PEEP, low tidal volume ventilation aims to minimize ventilator-associated lung injury due to volutrauma or atelectrauma. In severe ARDS with refractory hypoxemia, various specialized therapies and rescue strategies have been studied, including prone ventilation, NMBs, inhaled vasodilators, and ECMO. However, efficacy data are limited. Management of severe ARDS remains a challenge for clinicians.

Prone ventilation has been evaluated in many studies since the early 2000s. Those studies showed that prone ventilation improves oxygenation but offers no survival benefit (2). However, a subset of the population with severe refractory hypoxemia (Pao_2/Fio_2 ratio <100) did have a significant survival benefit. The finding was confirmed with a recent large randomized trial of early prone ventilation for severe ARDS (3). That study rejuvenated interest in prone ventilation. Oxygenation in the patient described above improved initially, but the effect was not lasting; refractory hypoxemia developed within days after the patient was transitioned to the supine position.

The use of NMBs in patients with severe ARDS has also been evaluated (4). A short-term (48-hour) continuous infusion of cisatracurium in the early phase of ARDS improved oxygenation, number of ventilator-free days, and 90-day survival without a difference in ICU-acquired neuromuscular weaknesses. Inhaled vasodilators are thought to improve ventilation-perfusion mismatch by improving oxygenation in the ventilated lung and relieving pulmonary hypertension. However, they improve oxygenation only transiently and are not known to provide a survival benefit (5).

The role of ECMO in patients with severe ARDS is still controversial. Previous studies did not show mortality benefit among patients with severe life-threatening hypoxemia. However, during the 2009-2010 H1N1 influenza A virus pandemic, ECMO was used as a rescue therapy in New Zealand and Australia. Studies from those countries reported 71% survival for ICU patients and a hospital discharge rate of 50% (6,7). A recent systematic review and meta-analysis showed variable outcomes among studies (8%-65%) (8). ECMO has a role for patients with severe ARDS, but further studies are needed to identify patients who would benefit from this resource-intensive therapy.

Oseltamivir and zanamivir are neuraminidase inhibitors that are effective against influenza A virus. Zanamivir is reserved for influenza virus strains known or suspected to be oseltamivir resistant. Its use in critically ill patients with severe ARDS has been shown to improve mortality, particularly when used within 5 days after symptom onset (9).

The evidence for high-dose oseltamivir therapy in influenza is limited. A multicenter double-blind randomized trial in Southeast Asia compared the use of double-dose oseltamivir (150 mg twice daily) with the standard dose (75 mg twice daily) in children and adults. No difference was found between the 2 groups in

ICU length of stay, duration of mechanical ventilation, clearance of virus, or mortality (10). The 2010 World Health Organization guideline recommended high doses of oseltamivir and longer duration of treatment of critically ill and immunocompromised patients even though data are lacking.

Severe influenza A–associated ARDS is difficult to manage, and supportive care is the cornerstone of treatment. To date, low tidal volume ventilation is the only proven strategy that improves mortality. Specialized therapies such as prone ventilation and ECMO are promising, but more randomized trials are needed to show survival benefit and define the best target population. The use of NMBs and inhaled vasodilators should be considered as adjunctive therapies. Neuraminidase inhibitors should be used early in the treatment of influenza A viral pneumonia.

REFERENCES

1. Putensen C, Theuerkauf N, Zinserling J, Wrigge H, Pelosi P. Meta-analysis: ventilation strategies and outcomes of the acute respiratory distress syndrome and acute lung injury. Ann Intern Med. 2009 Oct 20;151(8):566–76. Erratum in: Ann Intern Med. 2009 Dec 15;151(12):897.

2. Sud S, Friedrich JO, Taccone P, Polli F, Adhikari NK, Latini R, et al. Prone ventilation reduces mortality in patients with acute respiratory failure and severe hypoxemia: systematic review and meta-analysis. Intensive Care Med. 2010 Apr;36(4):585–99. Epub 2010 Feb 4.

3. Guerin C, Reignier J, Richard JC, Beuret P, Gacouin A, Boulain T, et al; PROSEVA Study Group. Prone positioning in severe acute respiratory distress syndrome. N Engl J Med. 2013 Jun 6;368(23):2159–68. Epub 2013 May 20.

4. Papazian L, Forel JM, Gacouin A, Penot-Ragon C, Perrin G, Loundou A, et al; ACURASYS Study Investigators. Neuromuscular blockers in early acute respiratory distress syndrome. N Engl J Med. 2010 Sep 16;363(12):1107–16.

5. Afshari A, Brok J, Moller AM, Wetterslev J. Inhaled nitric oxide for acute respiratory distress syndrome and acute lung injury in adults and children: a systematic review with meta-analysis and trial sequential analysis. Anesth Analg. 2011 Jun;112(6):1411–21. Epub 2011 Mar 3.

6. Davies A, Jones D, Bailey M, Beca J, Bellomo R, Blackwell N, et al; Australia and New Zealand Extracorporeal Membrane Oxygenation (ANZ ECMO) Influenza Investigators. Extracorporeal membrane oxygenation for 2009 influenza A (H1N1) acute respiratory distress syndrome. JAMA. 2009 Nov 4;302(17):1888–95. Epub 2009 Oct 12.

7. Peek GJ, Mugford M, Tiruvoipati R, Wilson A, Allen E, Thalanany MM, et al; CESAR trial collaboration. Efficacy and economic assessment of conventional ventilatory support versus extracorporeal membrane oxygenation for severe adult respiratory failure (CESAR): a multicentre randomised controlled trial. Lancet. 2009 Oct 17;374(9698):1351–63. Epub 2009 Sep 15. Erratum in: Lancet. 2009 Oct 17;374(9698):1330.

8. Zangrillo A, Biondi-Zoccai G, Landoni G, Frati G, Patroniti N, Pesenti A, et al. Extracorporeal membrane oxygenation (ECMO) in patients with H1N1 influenza infection: a systematic review and meta-analysis including 8 studies and 266 patients receiving ECMO. Crit Care. 2013 Feb 13;17(1):R30.

9. Louie JK, Yang S, Acosta M, Yen C, Samuel MC, Schechter R, et al. Treatment with neuraminidase inhibitors for critically ill patients with influenza A (H1N1)pdm09. Clin Infect Dis. 2012 Nov;55(9):1198–204. Epub 2012 Jul 26.

10. South East Asia Infectious Disease Clinical Research Network. Effect of double dose oseltamivir on clinical and virological outcomes in children and adults admitted to hospital with severe influenza: double blind randomised controlled trial. BMJ. 2013 May 30;346:f3039.

Severe Chest Pain

RONALDO A. SEVILLA BERRIOS, MD, AND R. THOMAS TILBURY, MD

CASE PRESENTATION

A 48-year-old man with a known history of hypertension with left ventricular hypertrophy, type 2 diabetes mellitus, and tobacco use presented to the emergency department with severe substernal chest pain. Pain was described as a constant substernal pressure. His initial electrocardiogram (ECG) showed nonspecific ST-T wave changes and mild diffuse ST-segment elevation similar to his previous ECGs. He was admitted for evaluation of possible acute coronary syndrome (ACS). Serial troponin levels were undetectable. His chest pain abated with morphine and lorazepam. Coronary computed tomography was planned for further evaluation of possible coronary artery disease. While in the hospital, the patient had severe substernal pain, described as 10 (on a scale from 0 to 10, with 10 being most severe), and marked pressure with radiation to the jaw and left arm. An ECG (Figure 49.1A) showed a new marked diffuse ST-segment elevation. After the patient was given aspirin and clopidogrel, he was taken to the cardiac catheterization laboratory emergently. Angiography (Figure 49.2) showed normal right and left coronary systems, and his ECG (Figure 49.1B) normalized after administration of morphine, nitroglycerin, and lorazepam intravenously.

The patient was transferred to the cardiac telemetry monitoring unit. Follow-up troponin levels remained undetectable, and he continued to be asymptomatic

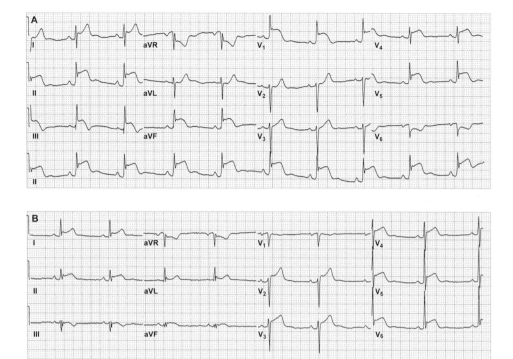

FIGURE 49.1. Electrocardiograms. A, At time of chest pain. B, Fifteen minutes later, after treatment with nitrates.

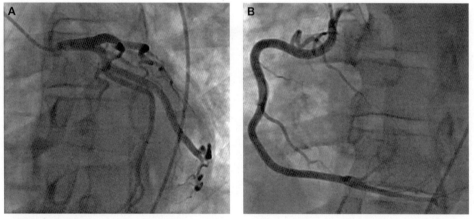

FIGURE 49.2. Angiograms. A, Left anterior oblique (LAO) view of left coronary artery. B, LAO view of right coronary artery.

after angiography. On further discussion, the patient admitted that he used cocaine while in the hospital 20 minutes before the episode of severe chest pain began. He was referred to the addiction service and instructed to follow up with the outpatient cardiology service.

DISCUSSION

ACS is a significant cause of morbidity and mortality in the United States (1). Prompt recognition and early revascularization have significantly decreased the frequency and severity of complications related to ACS (2). Several nonathero-sclerotic entities can resemble ACS and pose a challenge to physicians charged with the initial evaluation and triage of patients. The patient described above had nonatherosclerotic ACS with ECG changes suggestive of ST-segment elevation myocardial infarction (STEMI).

ACS consists of STEMI, non-STEMI, and unstable angina. ACS is a leading cause of emergency department visits in the United States. In patients with STEMI, timely revascularization with thrombolytics, early percutaneous cardiac intervention, or, when indicated, coronary artery bypass surgery is the mainstay of treatment with proven morbidity and mortality benefits (2). Treatment of non-STEMI is less defined, but the majority of patients are triaged toward evaluation with angiography.

Patients can present with chest pain from many conditions, such as aortic dissection, pneumonia, pulmonary embolism, pleuritis, gastroesophageal reflux or spasm, peptic ulcer disease, pancreatitis, costochondritis, rib fractures, or postherpetic neuralgia. Moreover, patients may present with ECG changes if they have myocarditis, acute pericarditis, stress-induced cardiomyopathy (ie, takotsubo cardiomyopathy), or coronary vasospasm induced by sympathomimetic agents.

Sympathomimetic or adrenergic stimulants can be associated with chest pain. Cocaine is one of the most common recreational drugs used worldwide, particularly among patients aged 18 to 45 years. The pathogenesis of cocaine-induced ischemia includes 1) an increased myocardial oxygen demand resulting from tachycardia and systemic hypertension and 2) a decreased oxygen supply resulting from coronary vasospasm. Cocaine also induces direct platelet activation, with the release of vasoactive granules causing thrombophilia and ischemic events. In patients with long-term cocaine use, it is not uncommon to find early atherosclerotic changes related to repetitive endothelial injury. Furthermore, cocaine use may be associated with other cardiovascular conditions, such as coronary artery aneurysm, myocarditis, and aortic dissection (3).

Patients with myocardial ischemia related to cocaine consumption present several unique treatment considerations. Early revascularization, antithrombotic strategies, and drug therapy continue to be the cornerstone for patients with coronary atherosclerosis. Coronary vasospasm is a major component in ACS related to cocaine. The use of β-blockers should be avoided in patients with acute cocaine intoxication because β-blockers may worsen coronary artery vasospasm and systemic hypertension secondary to unobstructed α-adrenergic stimulation in these patients (4). Nitroglycerin and calcium channel blockers are used preferentially and are effective for chest pain and hemodynamic stabilization. Benzodiazepines can be helpful by providing sedation, blood pressure control, and heart rate control during an acute episode. Finally, emphasis should be placed on secondary prevention by encouraging cocaine cessation, although this can be the most challenging step because it often requires a multidisciplinary team approach, including social support for long-term rehabilitation (5).

Cocaine is a commonly used illicit drug associated with significant cardiovascular complications, including ACS with coronary vasospasm. These syndromes may be difficult to differentiate from true plaque rupture and STEMI because their clinical and ECG presentations overlap. Early reperfusion and antiplatelet therapy may be used in both settings, although use of a β-blocker should be avoided in patients with cocaine intoxication. Nitrates, calcium channel blockers, and benzodiazepines are the preferred treatment.

REFERENCES

1. Murphy SL, Xu J, Kochanek KD. Deaths: preliminary data for 2010: National vital statistics reports; vol 60 no 4. Hyattsville (MD): National Center for Health Statistics; 2012.

2. Hochman JS, Sleeper LA, Webb JG, Sanborn TA, White HD, Talley JD, et al; for the SHOCK Investigators. Early revascularization in acute myocardial infarction complicated by cardiogenic shock. N Engl J Med. 1999 Aug 26;341(9):625–34.

3. Vasica G, Tennant CC. Cocaine use and cardiovascular complications. Med J Aust. 2002 Sep 2;177(5):260–2.

4. Fareed FN, Chan G, Hoffman RS. Death temporally related to the use of a Beta adrenergic receptor antagonist in cocaine associated myocardial infarction. J Med Toxicol. 2007 Dec;3(4):169–72.

5. Rezkalla SH, Kloner RA. Cocaine-induced acute myocardial infarction. Clin Med Res. 2007 Oct;5(3):172–6.

A More Frequent Airway Emergency

SHIHAB H. SUGEIR, MD,
AND FRANCIS T. LYTLE, MD

CASE PRESENTATION

A 79-year-old woman presented to the emergency department with severe swelling of her tongue. The swelling had progressed until she had difficulty swallowing her oral secretions. She reported that she had not been exposed to anything out of the ordinary. She was initially given epinephrine, methylprednisolone, and diphenhydramine, but she had little improvement in her symptoms. Her tongue swelling continued to worsen over the next hour such that airway compromise was a serious concern. An initial fiberoptic nasotracheal intubation performed by the emergency department resident was unsuccessful. The patient's airway was then secured with a fiberoptic orotracheal intubation by senior personnel from the anesthesia service. A review of the patient's history showed that this was the first incident of angioedema. She did not have any allergen exposures. Her medications included aspirin, labetalol, and lisinopril, none of which had been recently started or changed.

DISCUSSION

Laryngeal angioedema resulting from use of an angiotensin-converting enzyme inhibitor (ACEI) is a dangerous medical condition that can lead to significant morbidity and mortality. Of the patients presenting to hospitals with angioedema,

39% to 46% are taking an ACEI (1). Contributing to an increased frequency of ACEI-induced angioedema is the fact that stopping ACEI therapy does not seem to prevent the recurrence of angioedema (2). As more patients have received ACEI therapy, the incidence of angioedema and resultant difficult airway has increased. Thus, critical care providers must know what to do when a patient has ACEI-induced angioedema and a difficult airway.

To demystify and streamline decisions for managing a difficult airway, the American Society of Anesthesiologists has created an algorithm (Box 50.1 and Figure 50.1), which was recently updated (3). As outlined in the algorithm, several points should be addressed before attempting intubation (3): the cooperativeness of the patient, the ability to provide supplemental oxygenation, and the probable difficulty of mask ventilation.

The patient described above was cooperative, and supplemental oxygen was successfully administered by nasal cannula. Given the enlarged tongue, bag mask ventilation would be extraordinarily difficult or impossible. Therefore, the patient was maintained with spontaneous breathing during the awake intubation portion

---

BOX 50.1.
ALGORITHM FOR MANAGING A DIFFICULT AIRWAY, PART 1

1. Assess the likelihood and clinical impact of basic management problems
   - Difficulty with patient cooperation or consent
   - Difficult mask ventilation
   - Difficult supraglottic airway placement
   - Difficult laryngoscopy
   - Difficult intubation
   - Difficult surgical airway access

2. Actively pursue opportunities to deliver supplemental oxygen throughout the process of difficult airway management

3. Consider the relative merits and feasibility of basic management choices
   - Awake intubation vs intubation after induction of general anesthesia
   - Noninvasive technique vs invasive techniques for the initial approach to intubation
   - Video-assisted laryngoscopy as an initial approach to intubation
   - Preservation vs ablation of spontaneous ventilation

4. Develop primary and alternative strategies (see Figure 50.1)

Adapted from Apfelbaum et al (3). Used with permission.

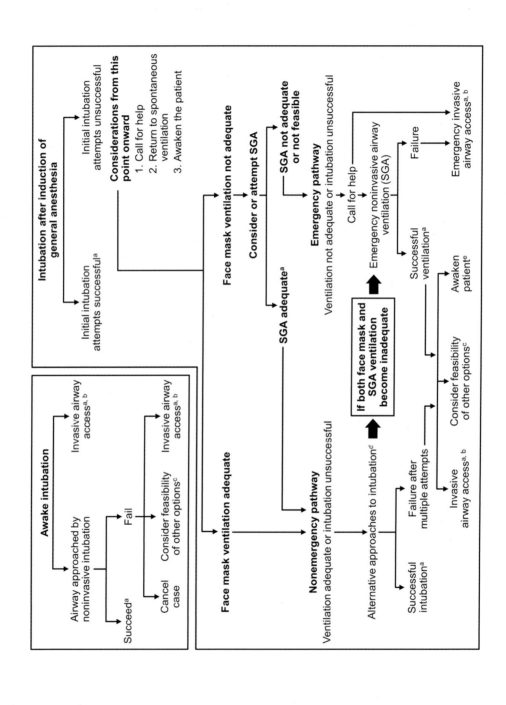

Awake intubation

Airway approached by noninvasive intubation

Succeed[a] → Cancel case

Succeed[a] → Invasive airway access[a, b]

Fail → Consider feasibility of other options[c]

Fail → Invasive airway access[a, b]

Intubation after induction of general anesthesia

Initial intubation attempts successful[a]

Initial intubation attempts unsuccessful

Considerations from this point onward
1. Call for help
2. Return to spontaneous ventilation
3. Awaken the patient

Face mask ventilation adequate

Nonemergency pathway
Ventilation adequate or intubation unsuccessful

Alternative approaches to intubation[d]

Successful intubation[a]

Failure after multiple attempts

Invasive airway access[a, b]

Consider feasibility of other options[c]

If both face mask and SGA ventilation become inadequate

Face mask ventilation not adequate

Consider or attempt SGA

SGA adequate[a]

SGA not adequate or not feasible

Emergency pathway
Ventilation not adequate or intubation unsuccessful

Call for help

Emergency noninvasive airway ventilation (SGA)

Successful ventilation[a]

Awaken patient[e]

Failure

Emergency invasive airway access[a, b]

FIGURE 50.1. Algorithm for Managing a Difficult Airway, Part 2. SGA indicates supraglottic airway. Footnotes indicate the following:

[a]Confirm ventilation, tracheal intubation, or SGA placement with exhaled carbon dioxide.

[b]Invasive airway access includes surgical or percutaneous airway, jet ventilation, and retrograde intubation.

[c]Other options include face mask or SGA anesthesia (eg, laryngeal mask airway [LMA], intubating LMA [ILMA], or laryngeal tube), local anesthesia infiltration, or regional nerve block. Pursuit of these options usually implies that mask ventilation will not be problematic. Therefore, these options may have limited value if this step has been reached through the emergency pathway.

[d]Alternative approaches include video-assisted laryngoscopy, alternative laryngoscope blades, SGA (eg, LMA or ILMA) as an intubation conduit (with or without fiberoptic guidance), fiberoptic intubation, intubating stylet or tube charger, light wand, and blind oral or nasal intubation.

[e]Consider preparing the patient for awake intubation or canceling the surgical procedure.

(Adapted from Apfelbaum et al [3]. Used with permission.)

of the difficult airway algorithm. When her airway was secured, she was sedated for comfort while the angioedema resolved over the following 48 hours.

Treatment of the patient described above provides positive and negative learning points. First, the difficulty of the initial airway was appreciated by the providers in the emergency department, and the patient was not cavalierly paralyzed for laryngoscopy (video or otherwise). Although videolaryngoscopy may be useful in mild or early angioedema, any manipulation of an already edematous airway will lead to further edema, with the potential for worsening the situation. Second, the request for help from the anesthesia service came too late. The call for help was after the failed attempt, when the airway was challenging because of increased edema and bleeding. Third, surgical backup was available. Although a surgical airway is not generally first-line therapy for a difficult airway, after the initial attempt failed, it would have been reasonable to have an experienced surgical team at the bedside. Finally, a difficult airway from angioedema may not be the best learning airway for inexperienced providers. Certainly this varies from patient to patient, but often the first attempt is the most likely to succeed, and having the most experienced provider attempt the airway first may be indicated (3).

REFERENCES

1. Rasmussen ER, Mey K, Bygum A. Angiotensin-converting enzyme inhibitor-induced angioedema: a dangerous new epidemic. Acta Derm Venereol. 2014 May;94(3):260-4.

2. Beltrami L, Zanichelli A, Zingale L, Vacchini R, Carugo S, Cicardi M. Long-term follow up of 111 patients with angiotensin-converting enzyme inhibitor-related angioedema. J Hypertens. 2011 Nov;29(11):2273-7.

3. Apfelbaum JL, Hagberg CA, Caplan RA, Blitt CD, Connis RT, Nickinovich DG, et al; American Society of Anesthesiologists Task Force on Management of the Difficult Airway. Practice guidelines for management of the difficult airway: an updated report by the American Society of Anesthesiologists Task Force on Management of the Difficult Airway. Anesthesiology. 2013 Feb;118(2):251-70.

Section II

Questions and Answers

Review Questions and Answers

QUESTIONS

Multiple Choice (choose the *best* answer)

1. Among the following, which is the most specific ultrasonographic sign of cardiac tamponade?
   a. Inferior vena cava dilatation
   b. Collapse of the inferior vena cava
   c. Systolic collapse of the right atrium
   d. Diastolic collapse of the right ventricle
   e. Circumferential pericardial effusion

2. A 56-year-old woman arrived in the emergency department with a 45-minute history of severe, substernal chest pain. The pain was described as pressure pain with an intensity of 10 (on a scale from 0-10, where 10 indicates the most severe pain) and radiating to her left arm and jaw. Her past medical history was significant for 60 pack-years of smoking, hypertension, and hypercholesterolemia. After she received initial treatment with oral aspirin and sublingual nitroglycerin, her reported pain level improved but persisted at an intensity of 5. On physical examination, her vital signs were heart rate 88 beats per minute, respiratory rate 19 breaths per minute, and blood pressure 95/64 mm Hg. She appeared distressed and diaphoretic. Cardiovascular and lung examination findings were unremarkable. An initial electrocardiogram showed new ST-segment elevation of 3 mm in leads II, III, and aVF.

The patient underwent cardiac catheterization and was found to have a severe occlusion of the right coronary artery. Direct balloon angioplasty and stent placement were successful. She was transferred to the intensive care unit in stable condition; 10 minutes later, her vital signs were heart rate 84 beats per minute, respiratory rate 18 breaths per minute, and blood pressure 88/56 mm Hg. Telemetry results are shown in Figure Q.2.

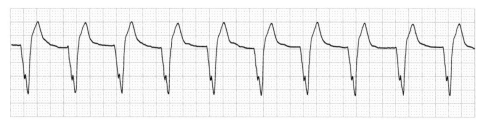

FIGURE Q.2. Telemetry Results.

What would be the next step?
a. Take her back to the cardiac catheterization laboratory because she is having a new infarct due to acute in-stent thrombosis
b. Give an additional dose of a β-blocker now
c. Sedate the patient for electrical cardioversion with 360 J from a biphasic defibrillator
d. Administer 1.0 L normal saline
e. Continue monitoring because the patient is hemodynamically stable

3. A 66-year-old man with a previous history of atrial fibrillation, hypertension, and obstructive sleep apnea has bradycardia and acutely elevated blood pressure accompanied by acute hypoxic respiratory failure after the reversal of anesthesia for bunion surgery. He undergoes emergent endotracheal intubation and receives mechanical ventilation. Multiple antihypertensive agents were required to control his blood pressure. As part of his evaluation, which of the following tests would likely provide the highest diagnostic yield?
a. Thyrotropin and free triiodothyronine
b. Serum and urine free metanephrines
c. Computed tomography of the chest, abdomen, and pelvis
d. Metaiodobenzylguanidine scan
e. Thyroid ultrasonography

TABLE Q8.1. Laboratory Test Results

Component	Result
Arterial blood gas	
pH	7.24
P_{CO_2}, mm Hg	24
P_{O_2}, mm Hg	98
Bicarbonate, mmol/L	18
Lactate, mmol/L	3.8
Glucose, mg/dL	118
Sodium, mmol/L	116
Chloride, mmol/L	84
Potassium, mmol/L	3.7
Lipase, U/L	784
Amylase, U/L	118
Aspartate aminotransferase, U/L	120
Alanine aminotransferase, U/L	56
Alkaline phosphatase, U/L	88
Triglycerides, mg/dL	4,890

The blood drawn in the emergency department was pink. You initiate fluid resuscitation (30 mL/kg), analgesics, and intravenous thiamine. What is the best next step in the management of this patient's disorder?

a. Administer 3% saline infusion

b. Initiate apheresis

c. Continue 0.9% saline, analgesia, and postpyloric nasogastric feeding

d. Perform computed tomography of the abdomen

e. Administer heparin infusion

9. A 28-year-old man with no relevant medical history presents to the hospital after 3 days of heavy alcohol consumption followed by severe emesis. In the emergency department, the patient was obtunded, with the following vital signs: heart rate 105 beats per minute, respiratory rate 34 breaths per minute, temperature 37.8°C, and blood pressure 110/72 mm Hg. Findings on the initial physical examination were unremarkable except for a fruity odor to his breath. Results of initial laboratory tests are shown in Table Q9.1.

TABLE Q9.1. Laboratory Test Results

Component	Result
Hematocrit, %	45
Leukocytes, ×10⁹/L	11
Sodium, mmol/L	149
Chloride, mmol/L	108
Bicarbonate, mmol/L	8
Serum urea nitrogen, mg/dL	45
Creatinine, mg/dL	1.2
Glucose, mg/dL	62
Albumin, g/dL	4
Arterial blood gas	
pH	7.28
$Paco_2$, mm Hg	18
Pao_2, mm Hg	309
Lactate, mmol/L	14.4
Serum osmolality, mOsm/kg	345
β-Hydroxybutyrate, mmol/L	3.1 (reference range <0.4)
Ethanol, mg/dL	165
Urine ketones	None

What is the most likely cause of this metabolic disarrangement?

a. Severe sepsis

b. Primary respiratory acidosis

c. Diabetic ketoacidosis

d. Alcohol-related euglycemic ketoacidosis

e. Methanol intoxication

10. A 19-year-old man with a history of major depression was brought to the hospital after he ingested more than 100 tablets of non–enteric-coated aspirin (325-mg tablets) in an attempt to end his life. He drank a glass of wine, but he denied ingesting other medications or drugs. Eight hours after aspirin ingestion, he felt scared and decided to seek medical attention. In the emergency department, he was awake, alert, and oriented. His Glasgow Coma Scale score was 15. Vital signs were blood pressure 115/70 mm Hg, pulse rate 86 beats per minute, respiration rate 10 breaths per minute, oxyhemoglobin saturation 98% on room air, and temperature 37.4°C. On physical examination, the

patient was not in respiratory distress. His cardiovascular, pulmonary, and gastrointestinal tract examinations were unremarkable. A spot blood glucose level was normal. The arterial blood gas results were pH 7.37, $Paco_2$ 41 mm Hg, and Pao_2 90 mm Hg at room air. Abdominal radiography did not show any radiopaque foreign bodies or tablets. Which of the following is *not* appropriate in the management of this patient?

a. Measure the salicylate level initially and then every 1 to 2 hours

b. Obtain results from a toxicology screen, including the acetaminophen level

c. Alkalinize the urine if the salicylate level is greater than 30 mg/dL

d. Give multiple doses of activated charcoal (25-50 g by mouth every 4 hours)

e. Admit the patient to a general ward because he is clinically stable 8 hours after ingestion

11. A 90-year-old woman with a history of hypertension is admitted to the hospital with an acute ST-segment elevation anterolateral wall myocardial infarction. She underwent urgent percutaneous coronary intervention with stenting of the left anterior descending artery. Persistent ST-segment elevation was noted on her 12-lead electrocardiogram after the procedure. Five days later, she had acute chest pain with diaphoresis and became profoundly hypotensive. Remarkable findings on physical examination were blood pressure 85/60 mm Hg, heart rate 120 beats per minute, respiratory rate 32 breaths per minute, oxygen saturation 91% with room air, and distended neck veins. Heart sounds were distant with no cardiac murmur, and her lungs were clear on auscultation. Which of the following is the most likely diagnosis?

a. Ruptured papillary muscles with acute mitral regurgitation

b. Rupture of the interventricular septum

c. Acute pericarditis with tamponade

d. Ventricular free wall rupture

e. Acute pulmonary embolism

12. A 35-year-old woman was admitted to the intensive care unit (ICU) after an episode of moderate hemoptysis. Her past medical history is significant for relapsed Hodgkin lymphoma. Three months ago, she underwent high-dose chemotherapy followed by autologous stem cell transplant. While in the ICU, she had another episode of massive hemoptysis and became unresponsive. Which of the following is the most appropriate next step?

a. Initiation of massive transfusion protocol

    b. Endotracheal intubation

    c. Administration of recombinant activated factor VII (rFVIIa)

    d. Urgent computed tomography of the chest

    e. Urgent bronchoscopy

13. According to the 9th edition of the American College of Chest Physicians guidelines, which of the following is an indication for systemic thrombolytic therapy in addition to anticoagulation, rather than anticoagulation alone, in the treatment of acute pulmonary embolism?

    a. Hypotension

    b. Right ventricular dysfunction

    c. Elevated troponin

    d. Age younger than 50 years

    e. Pleuritic chest pain

14. Which of the following statements best describes negative pressure pulmonary edema?

    a. It is characterized by negative intra-alveolar pressures

    b. It has been associated with upper airway obstruction

    c. It usually evolves over many hours

    d. It is treated with supplemental oxygen and diuretics

    e. Pulmonary hemorrhage has not been described as a complication

15. After left pneumonectomy, a 65-year-old man had severe hypotension, which was strongly suggestive of cardiac herniation. Preparations are being made to return the patient to the operating room to relieve the herniation. What can be done to minimize the hemodynamic perturbations related to his condition?

    a. Continue intravenous fluid volume resuscitation until the patient's hemodynamic condition improves

    b. Apply suction to the chest tube, and position the patient with the operative side down

    c. Arrange for extracorporeal membrane oxygenation

    d. Position the patient with the nonoperative side down, avoid hyperventilation of the lung, and return him to the operating room as soon as possible

    e. Observation

16. A 56-year-old man presents to the emergency department with fever, diminished vision, respiratory distress, and diffuse petechiae. Laboratory test

results include total leukocyte count 320×10^9/L, hemoglobin 5.8 g/dL, and platelet count 52×10^9/L. A chest radiograph shows diffuse bilateral airspace opacities. A peripheral blood smear shows 50% promyelocytes. Which of the following statements about this patient's blood tests is correct?

a. The plasma potassium result may be falsely low because of rapid metabolism by leukemic blasts

b. Automated platelet counts will be more accurate than manual counts because of the grossly elevated leukocyte count

c. The Pao$_2$ is more reliable than fingertip oxygen saturation

d. The plasma potassium result may be falsely elevated because of in vitro lysis of leukemic blasts

e. The hemoglobin result may be falsely low because of a dilutional effect from hyperleukocytosis

17. A 65-year-old man, a nonsmoker with no significant medical history and no family history of any cardiac disease, presented to the emergency department with chest pain. He rated the chest pain as 7 to 8 on a scale from 1 to 10 (10 indicating the most severe pain); it was substernal and nonradiating, with no relation to a change in position or to food intake. He reported that he had flulike symptoms 2 weeks before the chest pain, and he had been feeling weak with progressively worsening fatigue and dyspnea on exertion. He reported having had no contact with persons who were ill, he had no travel history, and he was not taking any new medications. On evaluation, he had tachycardia (heart rate 125 beats per minute), hypotension (blood pressure 85/60 mm Hg), jugular venous distention to 18 cm, and normal arterial oxygen saturation. On cardiac examination, the patient had an apical systolic murmur that did not have a thrill and did not change with dynamic maneuvers. He had a palpable, mildly tender liver but no edema or rash. Laboratory studies showed mild leukocytosis, normal levels of serum electrolytes, and normal renal and liver functions. He had mildly elevated cardiac troponin levels that did not increase significantly on serial measurements, mildly elevated creatine kinase MB isoform, but significantly elevated B-type natriuretic peptide. Electrocardiography showed sinus tachycardia, and chest radiography showed increased cardiothoracic diameter with prominent pulmonary vascular markings. Given these findings, what would you most likely expect to observe on a bedside transthoracic echocardiogram?

a. Global, severely reduced systolic function

b. Left ventricular outflow tract obstruction

c. Takotsubo cardiomyopathy

d. Acute coronary syndrome

e. Mural thrombus

18. A 58-year-old woman with metastatic ovarian cancer is transferred to the intensive care unit with acute onset of tachypnea, tachycardia, and hypotension. A chest radiograph obtained just before transfer shows an enlarged cardiac silhouette and bilateral moderate pleural effusions. The electrocardiogram shows beat-to-beat variability in QRS-complex amplitudes. What would you expect on physical examination and echocardiography? (Answer choices are described in Table Q18.1.)

TABLE Q18.1. Answer Choices With Examination and Echocardiographic Findings

Answer Choice	Physical Examination	Echocardiography
a.	Warm extremities, thready pulse, and mottling on the knees	Hyperdynamic left ventricle, inferior vena cava diameter 1.0 cm with inspiratory collapse >50%
b.	Pedal edema, palpable second heart sound in the left second intercostal space, and tender hepatomegaly	The right ventricle larger than the left ventricle, with bowing of the interventricular septum into the left ventricle and positive McConnell sign
c.	A high-pitched biphasic sound coinciding with the cardiac cycle and best audible at the lower left sternal border	Right atrial diastolic collapse lasting 25% of the cardiac cycle and a hypoechoic region posterior to the descending thoracic aorta on parasternal long-axis view
d.	A decrease in blood pressure by 12 mm Hg on inspiration and faint heart sounds	Right ventricular diastolic collapse and a hypoechoic region anterior to the descending thoracic aorta on parasternal long-axis view
e.	Jugular venous distention, a prominent third heart sound, and pedal edema	Four-chamber dilatation with hypoechoic material seen inside all cardiac chambers

19. A 57-year-old man with liver cirrhosis, septic shock, and acute kidney injury receives continuous renal replacement therapy with regional citrate anticoagulation. Which of the following laboratory test result sets may prompt you to decrease the citrate infusion rate? (Answer choices are described in Table Q19.1.)

TABLE Q19.1. **Answer Choices With Laboratory Test Results**

Answer Choice	Total Calcium, mg/dL	Ionized Calcium, mg/dL	Inorganic Phorphorus, mg/dL	Bicarbonate, mmol/L	Albumin, g/dL
a.	11.2	5.63	3.6	22	4.0
b.	10.8	3.60	4.6	17	3.5
c.	9.8	5.01	4.2	32	4.2
d.	7.8	4.09	2.6	12	3.6
e.	9.1	4.79	7.0	18	3.5

20. Which of the following is *not* associated with pituitary apoplexy?
    a. Hyperthyroidism
    b. Diabetes mellitus
    c. Sickle cell anemia
    d. Hypertension
    e. Head trauma

21. A 74-year-old man with congestive heart failure and asthma has been hospitalized after 3 days of fever and a worsening cough. In spite of receiving azithromycin, oseltamivir, and intravenous fluid boluses for hypotension, his respiratory status is deteriorating. Which of the following treatments would be appropriate?
    a. Continue oseltamivir orally for a total of 5 days
    b. Start methylprednisolone 1 mg/kg intravenously every 24 hours for influenza pneumonitis
    c. Discontinue broad-spectrum antibiotics if polymerase chain reaction is positive for influenza
    d. Start intravenous zanamivir for possible oseltamivir resistance
    e. None of the above is a recommended treatment strategy

22. A 69-year-old woman with a history of type 2 diabetes mellitus, treated breast cancer, and orthotopic liver transplant for autoimmune hepatitis is receiving mycophenolate mofetil, tacrolimus, and prednisone. She presented at the

hospital with dyspnea, cough, and a new rash that developed above her right eye and was followed by blisters. Chest radiography showed right lower and middle lobe pneumonia. Her condition quickly deteriorated, and she required intubation and mechanical ventilation. The skin lesions evolved rapidly, compromising the left eye and involving the ear lobes, maxillary areas, and right neck, with necrotic lesions in the nasal bridge and superior periorbital area. Blood cultures were started. In addition to a surgical consultation for débridement, which is the most appropriate next step in this patient's management?

a. Start broad-spectrum intravenous (IV) antibiotics

b. Start IV amphotericin B liposomal complex

c. Start broad-spectrum IV antibiotics and amphotericin B liposomal complex

d. Start IV caspofungin

e. Start broad-spectrum IV antibiotics and acyclovir

23. A 57-year-old woman actively undergoing treatment of metastatic pancreatic cancer is hospitalized with nausea, vomiting, and diarrhea. She suddenly becomes very light-headed and complains of feeling as if her heart is racing. A call for a rapid response team is activated; an electrocardiographic rhythm strip is shown in Figure Q.23.

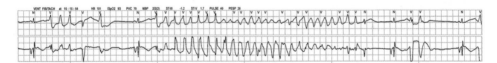

FIGURE Q.23. Electrocardiographic Rhythm Strip.

What is the priority of care for this patient?

a. Magnesium intravenously (IV)

b. Amiodarone IV

c. Adenosine IV

d. Lidocaine IV

e. Synchronized cardioversion

24. In patients with antiphospholipid antibody syndrome, which of the following tests would *not* be expected to be elevated?

a. Anticardiolipin antibody

b. Ferritin

c. β_2-Microglobulin

    d. Lupus anticoagulant

    e. Sedimentation rate

25. A 24-year-old man underwent laparotomy and debulking of a retroperitoneal sarcoma. Intraoperatively, he received 2 units of packed red blood cells and 3 L of lactated Ringer solution. Immediately after extubation in the operating room, stridor developed. After initial attempts at ventilation with an anesthesia bag and mask were unsuccessful, hypoxemia and bradycardia developed. Administration of atropine followed by propofol and succinylcholine restored airway patency, and subsequent positive pressure ventilation by mask improved oxygen saturation to 98%. In the postanesthesia care unit, however, hypoxemia recurred within a few minutes and required initiation of continuous positive airway pressure. Bilateral crackles were audible on chest auscultation, and chest radiography showed extensive bilateral pulmonary infiltrates. Which of the following is the most likely cause of the patient's condition?

    a. Transfusion-related acute lung injury (TRALI)

    b. Transfusion-associated circulatory overload (TACO)

    c. Aspiration-related acute lung injury

    d. Negative-pressure pulmonary edema

    e. Cardiogenic pulmonary edema due to perioperative myocardial infarction

26. A 23-year-old woman with type 1 diabetes mellitus presents with a 1-day history of nausea, vomiting, and abdominal pain. Because she has not been able to eat, she has been holding her insulin. Her heart rate is 140 beats per minute, and her blood pressure is 115/54 mm Hg. Results of laboratory investigations are shown in Table Q26.1.

TABLE Q26.1. **Laboratory Test Results**

Component	Result (Reference Range)
Sodium, mmol/L	135 (135–145)
Chloride, mmol/L	98 (100–108)
Bicarbonate, mmol/L	12 (22–29)
Potassium, mmol/L	3.3 (3.6–5.2)
Creatinine, mg/dL	0.9 (0.9–1.4)
Glucose, mg/dL	446 (70–140)
Urine ketones	4+
β-Hydroxybutyrate	Pending

Fluid boluses with normal saline are started and she is transferred to the intensive care unit. What is the most appropriate next step in her management?

a. Start an infusion of regular insulin

b. Obtain a computed tomographic scan of the abdomen and pelvis

c. Begin parenteral potassium replacement

d. Place an arterial line

e. Consult an endocrinology team

27. An 84-year-old woman with a history of progressive chronic lymphocytic leukemia (with bulky lymph nodes) was admitted for chemotherapy with dexamethasone and rituximab. Several hours after receiving rituximab, she had severe respiratory distress. Physical examination was remarkable for new atrial fibrillation with rapid ventricular response (heart rate 130 beats per minute), respiratory rate 30 breaths per minute, blood pressure 100/55 mm Hg, 100% oxygen saturation at 2 L/min, and splenomegaly. Laboratory test results showed marked acute leukopenia, hyperuricemia, hyperphosphatemia, hyperkalemia, acute kidney injury, and lactic acidosis. Chest radiography showed bilateral infiltrates and a right pleural effusion. What is the most likely cause of her acute kidney injury?

a. Cardiorenal syndrome caused by atrial fibrillation with rapid ventricular response

b. Rituximab-induced acute interstitial nephritis

c. Sepsis

d. Tumor lysis syndrome

e. Leukemia-induced interstitial nephritis

28. A 54-year-old woman with a history of Graves disease, hypertension, and diet-controlled diabetes mellitus was recently evaluated for acute worsening of chronic kidney disease and for new low-grade fevers and weight loss. Her urinalysis showed elevated protein, more than 100 red blood cells per high-power field, many dysmorphic red cells, and some red cell casts. On the day of her follow-up appointment, she had significant shortness of breath with a new cough, and she visited the emergency department. Vital signs were as follows: temperature 38°C, blood pressure 160/94 mm Hg, pulse 88 beats per minute, and oxygen saturation 83% with room air (corrected to 92% with oxygen delivered at 10 L/min through a face mask). She was pale and in moderate respiratory distress with bilateral

inspiratory crackles on lung examination. There was no peripheral edema. Chest radiography showed diffuse bilateral alveolar infiltrates. Results from an electrocardiogram were normal. Laboratory test results are shown in Table Q28.1.

TABLE Q28.1. **Laboratory Test Results**

Component	Result
Leukocyte count, ×10⁹/L	11.0
Differential leukocyte count	Within reference range
Hemoglobin, g/dL	7.1
Platelet count, ×10⁹/L	200
Creatinine, mg/dL	
Previous week	1.7
Present	4.5
Potassium, mmol/L	5.0
Erythrocyte sedimentation rate, mm/h	102
C-reactive protein, mg/L	132

Blood and sputum samples were drawn for cultures, and therapy was started with broad-spectrum antibiotics.

The patient now has refractory hypoxia requiring intubation and mechanical ventilation. Ventilation was set in the assist-control mode: tidal volume 6 mL/kg, respiratory rate 22 breaths per minute, positive end-expiratory pressure 15 mm Hg with peak pressure 30 mm Hg and plateau pressure 25 mm Hg, and 100% fraction of inspired oxygen resulting in oxygen saturations of 89%. An urgent bedside echocardiogram showed a hyperdynamic left ventricle (ejection fraction 75%), normal diastolic function, no valvular disease, and a completely collapsible inferior vena cava. Bronchoscopy showed bloody material in the upper lobes, and alveolar lavage produced a progressively blood-tinged return. Results for bacterial, viral, and fungal stains and cultures on the alveolar sample are pending. What should be done next?

a. Administer fresh frozen plasma

b. Place a central venous catheter and start plasmapheresis

    c. Administer methylprednisolone 1,000 mg intravenously (IV)

    d. Place a central venous catheter and start hemodialysis

    e. Administer furosemide 80 mg IV

29. What is the suspected mechanism associated with paraneoplastic neurologic syndromes?

    a. Direct effect of a tumor or cancer

    b. Direct effect of metastasis of a tumor or cancer

    c. Antibodies against antigens present in a tumor and the nervous system

    d. Metabolic derangement associated with malignancy

    e. Neuronal injury from cerebral edema

30. A 65-year-old woman with diet-controlled type 2 diabetes mellitus presents to the emergency department with a 3-day history of subjective chills; weakness; explosive, loose, watery, nonbloody stools; and abdominal pain 1 week after completing a 10-day course of oral clindamycin for a dental infection. Vital signs showed that she was febrile (38.6°C), tachycardic (heart rate 112 beats per minute), and hypotensive (blood pressure 86/62 mm Hg); her respiratory rate was 22 breaths per minute. On examination, her abdomen was tender. Polymerase chain reaction analysis of stool for *Clostridium difficile* toxin was positive. Radiography of the abdomen showed small-bowel ileus with no air under the diaphragm. Computed tomography of the abdomen showed extensive colonic wall thickening. The patient is hydrated, and intravenous metronidazole and oral vancomycin were initiated in the intensive care unit. Laboratory test results include the following: leukocyte count 31×10^9/L, creatinine 1.3 mg/dL (baseline 0.8 mg/dL), potassium 3.2 mmol/L, and serum lactate 2.4 mmol/L. Along with management for severe sepsis, with resuscitation and antibiotic therapy, which of the following additional interventions would be most beneficial at this time?

    a. Intravenous vancomycin

    b. Fecal microbiota transplantation

    c. Intravenous immunoglobulin administration

    d. Surgical consultation

    e. Oral fidaxomicin

31. A 6-year-old boy visiting Florida from Puerto Rico presents with a history of 4 days of fever, a petechial rash, and acute development of abdominal pain,

vomiting, and signs suggestive of shock. Encephalopathy and acute hypoxemic respiratory failure develop with a significant right-sided pleural effusion. The epidemiology, clinical picture, and laboratory results are suggestive of dengue hemorrhagic fever. In addition to intravenous fluids, what should be the recommended approach for this patient?

a. Vasoactive agents to maintain blood pressure, mechanical ventilation, and chest tube placement to drain the pleural effusion

b. Vasopressors and corticosteroids to maintain blood pressure, and mechanical ventilation for acute respiratory failure

c. Vasopressors to maintain blood pressure, and fresh whole blood for bleeding complications

d. Packed red blood cell transfusion for bleeding complications, and intravenous immunoglobulin to treat the underlying disease

e. Vasopressors to maintain blood pressure, and recombinant factor VII to correct coagulation abnormalities

32. A 50-year-old man was admitted to the intensive care unit from the emergency department for severe sepsis secondary to soft tissue infection. On further evaluation, he described recurrent high-grade fever for the past 3 months. He was admitted to another hospital 3 times during this period for similar complaints and was treated with intravenous antibiotics; his symptoms improved, but no definitive source of infection was found. He was morbidly obese and had taken prednisone for asthma since childhood. On examination, he looked anxious and his oral mucosa was dry. Examination of the heart, lungs, and abdomen was unremarkable. He had a localized soft tissue infection of the left lower leg and elbow. His laboratory test values at the time of admission to the intensive care unit included leukocytes 4.0×10^9/L, creatinine 1.7 mg/dL, sodium 135 mmol/L, and potassium 3.7 mmol/L. Which of the following test results would lead you to think of a diagnosis other than severe sepsis?

a. Elevated serum triglyceride level

b. Profoundly elevated serum ferritin level

c. Bone marrow biopsy with evidence of erythrophagocytosis

d. Leukopenia

e. All of the above

33. A 66-year-old man with a history of cirrhosis secondary to nonalcoholic fatty liver disease complicated by esophageal varices and hepatic encephalopathy is admitted to the intensive care unit for acute infection with influenza virus; he is intubated upon arrival. Because of significant abdominal distention, a diagnostic paracentesis is performed, and ascitic fluid analysis shows a total nucleated cell count of 670/mcL with 56% neutrophils; however, ascitic fluid cultures remain negative. Which of the following is the best next step in treatment of this patient?

    a. Repeat the diagnostic paracentesis and send a fluid sample for microbiology testing

    b. Initiate cefotaxime therapy

    c. Do not initiate antibiotic therapy yet because the cultures are negative

    d. Initiate diuretic therapy with furosemide and spironolactone

    e. Begin evaluation for liver transplant

34. A 35-year-old man from Southeast Asia who had a past history of untreated hepatitis B virus infection presented to the emergency department with a history of 2 weeks of fatigue, malaise, intermittent fever associated with nausea, and bilateral flank pain. He did not have diarrhea, rash, gross hematuria, or urinary tract symptoms. Two days before presentation, he noticed difficulties in walking due to right foot drop. On examination and testing, he had accelerated hypertension (190/110 mm Hg), leukocytosis, elevated creatinine level, microscopic hematuria, and mild proteinuria with an absence of dysmorphic erythrocytes. He had normal liver function test results, but elevated values for erythrocyte sedimentation rate and C-reactive protein. He was admitted to the intensive care unit for management of accelerated hypertension and acute kidney injury. Further tests showed normal results for antinuclear antibody, antineutrophil cytoplasmic autoantibody, C3, and C4 and negative results for anti–glomerular basement membrane antibody, hepatitis C virus, human immunodeficiency virus, and cryoglobulin. Ultrasonography showed kidneys of normal size but with multiple wedge-shaped infarctions. Renal angiography showed multiple microaneurysms of the renal artery bilaterally but no evidence of dissection. What is the most likely cause of this patient's hypertension and renal failure?

    a. Fibromuscular dysplasia

    b. Polyarteritis nodosa (PAN)

c. Cryoglobulinemia

d. Henoch-Schönlein purpura (immunoglobulin A–associated vasculitis)

e. Idiopathic renal artery dissection

35. A 63-year-old woman presents with hypoxic respiratory failure from aspiration pneumonia and septic shock. She is quickly intubated and successfully managed with fluids, antibiotics, and vasopressors. On day 4 of her stay in the intensive care unit, her sedation is stopped and she is found to be diffusely weak and she cannot be successfully weaned from mechanical ventilation. On examination, she has a third cranial nerve palsy on the right side, bifacial weakness, a flaccid quadraparesis, and diffuse areflexia. Her serum creatine kinase level is normal, and nerve conduction studies show a reduction in the compound muscle action potential (CMAP) and sensory nerve action potential amplitudes with prolonged conduction velocities. Which of the following is *not* consistent with the diagnosis of critical illness neuromyopathy?

a. Areflexia

b. Flaccid quadraplegia

c. Normal creatine kinase

d. Reduced CMAP amplitudes on nerve conduction study

e. Third cranial nerve palsy on the right side

36. A 43-year-old woman with a history of bipolar disorder (treated with lithium and quetiapine) and migraine headaches receives prochlorperazine from her primary physician for treatment of a migraine exacerbation. Despite multiple doses, her headache does not improve and her husband brings her to the emergency department because she has become progressively confused and lethargic since taking the medication. On presentation, she is stuporous and febrile with normal pupils and diffuse rigidity. She is using accessory respiratory muscles and has a limited ability to expand her chest with air. Red urine is apparent in her Foley catheter drainage bag. Her temperature is 42.1°C, her blood pressure is 196/103 mm Hg, her heart rate is 135 beats per minute, and her respiratory rate is 33 breaths per minute, with an oxygen saturation of 91% with room air. Arterial blood gas studies show pH 6.9, Pao_2 61 mm Hg, and $Paco_2$ 69 mm Hg. What is the most appropriate next step?

a. Immediately administer intravenous (IV) dantrolene

b. Immediately administer bicarbonate for renal protection

c. Immediately administer bromocriptine

    d. Perform endotracheal intubation

    e. Administer 30 mg IV labetalol

37. A 36-year-old woman who takes levothyroxine for hypothyroidism and who has a remote history of binge alcohol use presented to the emergency department with a 36-hour history of nausea, vomiting, sweating, and weakness. Her boyfriend reported that during an argument 2 days ago, she threatened to end her life. She was lethargic, oriented, afebrile, tachycardic (heart rate 116 beats per minute), and hypotensive (blood pressure 88/58 mm Hg), and her respiratory rate was 17 breaths per minute. On physical examination, she had right upper quadrant tenderness without peritoneal signs. A computed tomographic scan of the abdomen was unremarkable. Laboratory test results included the following: aspartate aminotransferase 2,100 U/L, alanine aminotransferase 2,450 U/L, bilirubin 2.2 mg/dL, glucose 45 mg/dL, international normalized ratio 2.3, and serum ammonia 124 mcmol/L. Along with resuscitation and stabilization as appropriate, which would be the best next step in the management of this patient?

    a. Administer cimetidine

    b. Administer *N*-acetylcysteine

    c. Obtain serum acetaminophen levels

    d. Administer lactulose

    e. Obtain serum ethanol levels

38. Which of the following is *not* associated with hepatic encephalopathy?

    a. Hyperreflexia

    b. Muscle rigidity

    c. Focal neurologic deficit

    d. Decerebrate posturing

    e. Reversibility with bicarbonate

39. A 72-year-old woman has a previous history of coronary artery disease, atrial fibrillation (she receives warfarin therapy), hypertension, chronic alcohol use, drug abuse, and diabetes mellitus. She presents with obtundation after a witnessed fall from standing height. She is emergently intubated with midazolam and vecuronium and brought to the local emergency department. Neurologic examination shows an absence of motor response and an absence of all brainstem reflexes with the exception of a repetitive stereotypical foot

dorsiflexion response to foot stimulation. Computed tomography of the head shows a large left frontotemporal hemorrhage with subfalcine, uncal, and tonsillar herniation. Her temperature is 33°C. The physician proceeds to perform an apnea test and declares that she is brain-dead. Which of the following statements is true?

a. Metabolic abnormalities and alcohol were not ruled out as potential confounders

b. Brain death was declared inappropriately because the patient had a foot dorsiflexion response to foot stimulation

c. The patient did not need to be warmed to normothermia before the neurologic examination

d. Adequate time was allowed for the clearance of medications she received during intubation

e. Brain death requires an ethics consultation before final declaration

40. When initiating extracorporeal membrane oxygenation (ECMO) therapy for acute hypoxic respiratory failure in a critically ill adult, which of the following statements is correct?

a. Neuromuscular blockade should be continued for as long as the patient receives ECMO

b. Mechanical ventilation is not necessary for any patient receiving venoarterial ECMO

c. Venovenous ECMO is the initial therapy of choice for patients with isolated, severe hypoxic respiratory failure

d. Antimicrobial prophylaxis has been proved to reduce the risk of central line–associated infections with ECMO

e. The recommended time for ECMO initiation is after a minimum of 7 to 10 days of conventional mechanical ventilation

41. A 42-year-old man with a long-standing history of intravenous drug abuse presents with sudden-onset hypoxemic respiratory failure and requires endotracheal intubation. Chest radiography shows normal cardiac silhouette size and bilateral diffuse infiltrates consistent with pulmonary edema. Which of the following is most likely to aid in making the definitive diagnosis?

a. Physical examination

b. Electrocardiography

  c. Echocardiography

  d. Cardiac catheterization

  e. Computed tomography of the chest

42. An 82-year-old man with a history significant for hyperlipidemia, peripheral vascular disease, and severe coronary artery disease is admitted to the intensive care unit with severe abdominal pain, hypotension, and an elevated lactate concentration (4.5 mmol/L). He has recently undergone celiac artery stent replacement for arterial stenosis. A plain radiograph of the abdomen shows intramural gas in the intestinal mucosa. After initial fluid resuscitation is started, what is the best next step of action?

  a. Perform a computed tomographic scan of the abdomen with a contrast agent to examine the visceral vasculature for patency

  b. Perform a full abdominal ultrasonographic examination of the abdomen to examine blood flow to the visceral organs

  c. Continue symptomatic support and observe the patient for improvement

  d. Arrange for the patient to return to the operating room for surgical exploration

  e. Arrange for colonoscopy

43. A 59-year-old man presented with neutropenic fever, fatigue, rash, and marked diarrhea 9 days after autologous stem cell transplant for multiple myeloma. At admission, he was profoundly neutropenic with a leukocyte count of 0.1×10^9/L. An infectious disease workup, broad-spectrum antimicrobials, and intravenous fluid repletion were begun. Blood, sputum, and urine cultures were negative for growth. Chest radiography did not show any infiltrate. Over the next 4 days, although his leukocyte count increased to 1.3×10^9/L, his clinical status deteriorated. Worsening dyspnea, hypoxia, and oliguria developed, necessitating transfer to the intensive care unit. Portable chest radiography showed new bilateral interstitial infiltrates. Electrocardiographic and troponin results were normal. Which is the most appropriate next step in management?

  a. Administer methylprednisolone

  b. Administer furosemide

  c. Perform bronchoalveolar lavage

  d. Perform a lung biopsy

  e. Continue current management

44. A 36-year-old man presents to the emergency department after a motor vehicle accident in which he was the unrestrained driver in a head-on collision with another car. His heart rate is 98 beats per minute, his blood pressure is 130/85 mm Hg, his respiratory rate is 28 breaths per minute, his oxygen saturation is 86% while breathing oxygen delivered at 6 L/min by nasal cannula, and his Glasgow Coma Scale score is 15. His voice is clear, he can speak in short phrases, and he reports chest pain. On examination he has a midline trachea, nondistended neck veins, anterior chest wall bruising, and equal breath sounds with crackles over the right anterior chest. His abdomen is flat, soft, and nontender. His pelvis is stable. His extremities are warm with normal distal pulses, normal capillary refill time, and no indication of a long-bone fracture. A chest radiograph shows an infiltrate in the right mid lung field. No rib fractures are seen. The mediastinum and cardiac silhouette are not enlarged. In addition to endotracheal intubation, which of the following is appropriate for this patient?

    a. Insert a right-sided chest tube

    b. Perform computed tomographic (CT) angiography of the chest to confirm aortic dissection

    c. Administer broad-spectrum antibiotics, including anaerobic coverage for aspiration pneumonitis

    d. Avoid giving excessive intravenous fluids, and perform CT of the chest

    e. Perform pericardiocentesis

45. Which is true for thyroid replacement in patients with myxedema?

    a. Myxedema coma should be corrected slowly to avoid seizures

    b. Triiodothyronine (T_3) is preferred to thyroxine (T_4) because it has a more gradual onset of action

    c. Even in the presence of myxedema ileus, oral doses of T_4 have been reported to provide excellent clinical responses

    d. T_3 is peripherally converted to T_4

    e. The appropriate dose of thyroid hormone replacement has not been well established

46. You are evaluating an 81-year-old man for persistent anemia, easy bruising, and urologic bleeding. He has no personal or family history of a bleeding

disorder. You suspect an acquired factor inhibitor. Which of the following would *not* aid in the diagnosis of factor inhibitors?

a. Prothrombin time

b. Bleeding time

c. Activated partial thromboplastin time

d. Mixing study

e. Genetic testing for specific mutations

47. A previously healthy 32-year-old man is seen in the emergency department for blunt chest wall trauma after a motor vehicle accident. He is tachycardic (heart rate 120 beats per minute), tachypneic (respiration rate 32 breaths per minute), and complaining of chest pain. His blood pressure is 87/45 mm Hg. His oxygen saturation is 92% while breathing 100% oxygen from a nonre-breather mask. Breath sounds are diminished but present. A bedside lung ultrasonogram from the left anterior chest is shown in Figure Q.47.

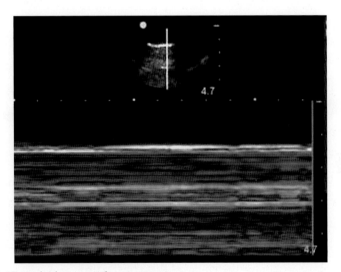

FIGURE Q.47. Bedside Lung Ultrasonogram.

What is the next appropriate step?

a. Noninvasive mechanical ventilation

b. Needle thoracostomy

c. Pericardiocentesis

d. Bronchoscopy

e. Chest radiography

48. Which of the following statements is true about management of patients who have severe influenza-associated acute respiratory distress syndrome (ARDS)?

a. Prone ventilation is recommended as routine therapy for severe ARDS

b. The use of extracorporeal membrane oxygenation therapy is most beneficial in the fibroproliferative phase of ARDS

c. Double-dose oseltamivir therapy with longer duration is recommended for critically ill or immunocompromised patients

d. Continuous infusion of a neuromuscular blocker transiently improves refractory hypoxemia

e. The use of inhaled vasodilators results in long-lasting resolution of hypoxemia

49. A 65-year-old woman who presents with chest pain has a history significant for hypertension, hyperlipidemia, and an ischemic cerebrovascular accident and ischemic stroke 2 years ago that left her with mild weakness in her left lower extremity. She had an ST-segment elevation myocardial infarction 1 month ago that was treated with percutaneous coronary stenting in the mid right coronary artery. She was improving until 6 hours ago, when substernal chest pain developed. The chest pain is worse with inspiration and coughing, is relieved by leaning forward, and is associated with mild shortness of breath and a low-grade fever. She reports no palpitations or syncope. Physical examination findings were significant for auscultation of a scratching sound throughout the cardiac cycle. The patient took ibuprofen with partial improvement of her symptoms 2 hours earlier. The initial electrocardiogram at presentation in the emergency department showed normal sinus rhythm; Q waves in leads II, III, and aVF; and diffuse ST-segment elevation. What is the best explanation for the cause of this chest pain?

a. Myocardial interstitium with abundant edema and an inflammatory infiltrate with lymphocytes and macrophages

b. Autoimmune antibody–mediated inflammatory process targeting cardiac antigens

c. Endovascular rupture of fibrous plaque with a proteoglycan matrix and lipid-laden cells exposing the underlying necrotic core and allowing thrombus formation

d. Significant reduction in nitric oxide synthase–containing neurons, inducing impaired relaxation

e. Mechanical dysfunction of the costotransverse joint

50. A 54-year-old man was recently prescribed lisinopril for poorly controlled hypertension. Approximately 1 week after starting his medication, he awoke with swelling of his lower lip. He presented to the emergency department several hours later with increased swelling of his lower lip and tongue. He is having difficulty talking but can adequately oxygenate. His ability to protect his airway became a concern after he did not have a response to diphenhydramine and epinephrine. You attempt rapid-sequence intubation, but you cannot visualize the vocal cords. Oxygen saturation by pulse oximetry is 80% and decreasing. What should your next step be?

a. Reposition the patient, change from a Miller blade to a MacIntosh blade, and try direct laryngoscopy again

b. Attempt placement of a supraglottic airway, such as a laryngeal mask airway

c. Call for help, and provide supplemental oxygenation with a bag mask

d. Attempt to create a surgical airway, such as a needle cricothyrotomy

e. Attempt a videolaryngoscopic intubation

ANSWERS

1. Answer d.

Cardiac tamponade occurs when pressure within the pericardial space exceeds the pressure in the cardiac chambers and impedes filling of the heart. Inferior vena cava plethora (choice *a*) is a very sensitive sign for cardiac tamponade, but it lacks specificity and so is less helpful in ruling in the diagnosis when seen ultrasonographically (J Am Coll Cardiol. 1988 Dec;12[6]:1470-7). Collapse of the inferior vena cava (choice *b*) would make cardiac tamponade less likely because inferior vena cava plethora is a very sensitive finding in cardiac tamponade. Diastolic collapse of the right atrium (not systolic collapse, as in choice *c*) is a moderately sensitive (55%) and highly specific (88%) finding (J Am Coll Cardiol. 1988 Dec;12[6]:1470-7). The right atrium is a thin-walled structure, and a brief collapse of the right atrial wall can occur in the absence of cardiac tamponade. If the duration of right atrial diastolic collapse exceeds one-third of the cardiac cycle, it is nearly 100% sensitive and specific for tamponade (J Am Soc Echocardiogr. 2013 Sep;26[9]:965-1012.e15). Early diastolic collapse of the right ventricle (choice *d*) signifies that the pericardial pressure exceeds the right ventricular diastolic pressure, and it is a highly specific (95%) sign of cardiac tamponade (J Am Soc Echocardiogr. 2013 Sep;26[9]:965-1012.e15). It is generally accompanied by a 20% decrease in cardiac output (J Am Soc Echocardiogr. 2013 Sep;26[9]:965-1012.e15). Circumferential pericardial effusion (choice *e*) can be present with or without cardiac tamponade and, by itself, does not help confirm the diagnosis of cardiac tamponade.

2. Answer e.

This is an accelerated idioventricular rhythm that originated in the ventricle and is characterized by wide complexes with a rate of 60 to 100 beats per minute. It is frequently related to reperfusion and is present early after resolution of myocardial injury. It is usually a self-limited rhythm and does not need any intervention other than continued monitoring.

Choice *a* is wrong because the patient is not having a new infarct and does not need further intervention. Choice *b* is wrong because a β-blocker in this acute phase may inhibit the ventricular intrinsic rhythm, unmasking an underlying atrioventricular blockage and making the patient hemodynamically unstable. These types of arrhythmias are frequent when patients have ischemic changes in the right coronary artery system because the sinus node and the atrioventricular node are supplied by this artery. Generally, normal conduction is reestablished in the first 24 hours after the event, although some patients need a pacemaker.

Choices *c* and *d* are wrong because there is no need for immediate defibrillation or a bolus of fluids in a hemodynamically stable patient. Moreover, the dosing and modality of cardioversion and defibrillation are wrong. Monophasic defibrillation is no longer recommended because evidence has shown that biphasic energy is better for terminating ventricular tachycardia or ventricular fibrillation.

3. Answer b.

According to current evidence (Pancreas. 2010 Aug;39[6]:775-83), measurements of fractionated metanephrines (ie, normetanephrine and metanephrine measured separately) in urine or plasma provide superior diagnostic sensitivity over measurement of the parent catecholamines. Elevation of plasma metanephrines of more than 4-fold above the upper reference limit is associated with nearly 100% probability of the tumor. Therefore, measuring blood and urine levels of these metabolites in symptomatic patients has high diagnostic yield.

4. Answer a.

Progressive malaise, fatigue, and hepatomegaly with a cholestatic pattern is the typical presentation with amyloid liver involvement. Acute hepatitis (choice *b*), hemolysis (choice *c*), and isolated single-organ disease (choice *d*) are not associated with amyloid.

5. Answer d.

Severe blastomycosis is treated with amphotericin B deoxycholate or amphotericin B lipid complex intravenously until the patient shows clinical improvement; then itraconazole is given orally for 6 to 12 months. The use of systemic corticosteroids can also be considered if patients have acute respiratory distress syndrome associated with blastomycosis.

6. Answer e.

The clinical course, history of environmental exposure, and elevated eosinophils on bronchoalveolar lavage (BAL) are suggestive of acute eosinophilic pneumonia. Patients with Churg-Strauss syndrome are unlikely to present with respiratory failure without other systemic features (ie, upper airway disease, skin lesions, arthralgia, or renal involvement), and they usually have refractory or steroid-dependent asthma. Hypersensitivity pneumonitis can be triggered by inhalation of organic antigens, and patients present with recurrent, self-limited episodes of pneumonitis with a lymphocyte (and rarely neutrophil) predominance on BAL. Diffuse alveolar hemorrhage occurs in patients with connective tissue diseases (eg, lupus or small-vessel vasculitides), hemoptysis, and severe respiratory failure. Chest radiography usually shows bilateral infiltrates. The diagnosis is based on the presence of a bloody BAL return or abundant hemosiderin-laden macrophages.

7. Answer b.

The most likely cause in this scenario is menstrual toxic shock syndrome. This disease is typically mediated by *Staphylococcus aureus*, but the single most important aspect of care is source control. Therefore, conducting a gynecologic examination and removing tampons or other foreign materials is the most important first step. Although the antibiotics in choice *a* would be appropriate empirical therapy, this is not the most important first step, and the need for antibiotic therapy in menstrual toxic shock syndrome with adequate source control is questionable. There is no evidence that a transfusion is needed. Corticosteroids are not indicated in most cases of toxic shock syndrome—and certainly not as initial therapy. Thrombotic thrombocytopenic purpura (TTP) is unlikely in the absence of underlying pathology (eg, malignancy), and the normal values for hemoglobin and lactate dehydrogenase strongly argue against TTP. Furthermore, if TTP were suspected, a peripheral smear should be examined to look for schistocytes and fragmented erythrocytes before initiation of plasmapheresis.

8. Answer b.

The clinical scenario describes a case of severe acute pancreatitis in a patient with severe hypertriglyceridemia. Even with alcohol use, severe triglyceridemia can exist as a concomitant cause of acute pancreatitis and should be treated aggressively. Early initiation of apheresis is the treatment of choice. The sodium level of 116 mmol/L is likely a result of pseudohyponatremia related to severe hypertriglyceridemia and does not need to be treated separately until the triglyceride levels are corrected. Continuing 0.9% saline, analgesia, and postpyloric nasogastric feeding are all components of treating acute pancreatitis, but a more definitive aggressive approach for this patient would be to correct the hypertriglyceridemia. Computed tomography of the abdomen is not indicated initially for acute pancreatitis with no clinical signs of necrosis or hemorrhage.

Because of the transient action of heparin and the risk of bleeding, the use of heparin is controversial, and it should not be used as first-line therapy when apheresis is available.

9. Answer d.

This patient presented with alcohol-related ketoacidosis, which is induced typically by a period of starvation and heavy alcohol intake followed by severe vomiting. The ketosis is thought to result from depleted hepatic glycogen stores and increased sympathetic activity, which can occur without diabetes mellitus but is more common in diabetic patients. Alcoholic ketoacidosis occurs more frequently with hypoglycemia instead of hyperglycemia. This phenomenon is caused by inhibition of hepatic gluconeogenesis after depletion of the reduced form of nicotinamide adenine dinucleotide due to alcohol metabolism to acetate. The generation of ketones is mostly due to starvation with selective conversion of acetate to ketone bodies as a source of adenosine triphosphate.

10. Answer e.

Salicylate levels should be monitored frequently to ensure that they are decreasing. Patients with drug overdose commonly ingest multiple medications; therefore, a toxicology screen including over-the-counter medications such as salicylate and acetaminophen should be performed. Alkalinization of urine is recommended until the salicylate level is less than 30 mg/dL. This should be guided by urine pH. In addition, treatment with multiple doses of activated charcoal is appropriate beyond 2 hours after ingestion because of the large dose and the potential for ingestion of a delayed-release formulation. Therefore, this patient should be closely monitored in the intensive care unit until a downward trend in the salicylate level is confirmed.

11. Answer d.

Acute rupture of papillary muscles with mitral regurgitation typically develops in patients with inferior myocardial infarction who present clinically with a new holosystolic murmur, cardiogenic shock, and acute pulmonary edema. In the presence of a pulmonary artery catheter, a large *v* wave is usually seen on pulmonary capillary wedge tracing. Patients with rupture of the interventricular septum usually have a large anterior wall infarction and clinical findings similar to those described for ruptured papillary muscles. However, in the presence of a pulmonary artery catheter (in addition to a large *v* wave), a step-up in oxygenation from the right atrium to the right ventricle is diagnostic (the result of a left-to-right shunt through a ventricular septal defect). In addition, ventricular septal defects are commonly associated with a palpable thrill, which is uncommon with ruptured papillary muscles. The absence of pulmonary edema and a holosystolic murmur strongly argues against these 2 possibilities. The patient described in the question has features of pericardial tamponade. However, the sudden development of tamponade after chest pain points to a possible free wall rupture as a cause. Patients with acute, massive pulmonary embolism may present with obstructive shock, but embolism would not explain the tamponade features. Also, with obstructive shock due to massive embolism, significant hypoxemia would be expected.

12. Answer b.
Although this patient may need more than 1 intervention, endotracheal intubation should be the primary intervention. A large endotracheal tube (internal diameter ≥8 mm) should be used to ensure adequate suction and to facilitate interventions such as bronchoscopy. Resuscitation with fluids, blood, and blood products (to correct any preexisting coagulopathy) should be done as soon as the airway has been secured.

Although it is tempting to consider administering recombinant activated factor VII (rFVIIa) for massive hemoptysis, most experience with its use is anecdotal and, therefore, rFVIIa should be considered a salvage therapy. For patients in stable condition, computed tomography of the chest can be performed to help determine the site and cause of hemoptysis, especially if bronchoscopy is not readily available. Bronchoscopy is an important tool that can be used to determine the bleeding site, protect the unaffected lung, and stop the bleeding. However, bronchoscopy should be performed only after the airway has been protected and the patient is hemodynamically stable.

13. Answer a.
The 2012 (9th edition) American College of Chest Physicians (ACCP) guidelines recommend the administration of systemic thrombolytic therapy in patients with massive pulmonary embolism, provided there are no contraindications. These ACCP guidelines do not explicitly recommend systemic thrombolytics for patients with submassive pulmonary embolism with right ventricular dysfunction or elevated troponin.

14. Answer b.

Negative pressure pulmonary edema has been associated with upper airway obstruction. The rest of the statements are not true.

15. Answer d.

To stabilize the patient's condition while preparing for his return to the operating room, and in addition to providing vasopressor support as needed, conservative measures include positioning the patient with the nonoperative side down, avoiding hyperventilation of the other lung, and injecting air into the empty hemithorax.

16. Answer d.

The question describes a patient with acute promyelocytic leukemia presenting with leukostasis (symptomatic hyperleukocytosis). Laboratory test results for patients with leukostasis must be interpreted with caution. In vitro lysis of leukemic blasts or their rupture during transport, especially in pneumatic tube systems, may cause spurious hyperkalemia. Thus, answer choice *d* is correct and, by consequence, choice *a* is incorrect. Automated platelet counts may be spuriously elevated because of blast fragments being counted as platelets; hence, a manual platelet count will be more accurate (choice *b* is incorrect). Leukemic blasts rapidly consume the available oxygen in an arterial blood gas sample and can lead to a falsely low Pao_2 (choice *c* is incorrect). Spuriously low hemoglobin readings due to hyperleukocytosis have not been described in the literature (choice *e* is incorrect).

17. Answer a.

The most likely observation would be a profound decrease in cardiac function. This is supported by the history, which suggests a viral prodrome, and the elevated cardiac biomarkers and the imaging, which show increased pulmonary vascular markings suggestive of increased left ventricular diastolic pressures. Left ventricular outflow tract obstruction is less likely because of the absence of dynamic findings on auscultation. Takotsubo cardiomyopathy, although on the differential diagnosis, is difficult to predict without further investigations; it remains a diagnosis of exclusion. Acute coronary syndrome should always be in the differential diagnosis in a patient presenting with chest pain; however, in this instance the troponin levels were only mildly elevated without significant changes over serial measurements, which would make an acute coronary syndrome less likely.

However, heart failure secondary to a late presentation of myocardial infarction remains in the differential diagnosis. Of all the possible answers, global reduction in systolic function would be the finding most likely observed.

18. Answer d.

The question describes a case of cardiac tamponade in a patient with metastatic ovarian malignancy who has hemodynamic instability with electrical alternans. Answer choice *d* is the only one consistent with cardiac tamponade because the physical examination findings include pulsus paradoxus and muffled heart sounds, and echocardiography shows right ventricular diastolic collapse and pericardial effusion, seen as a hypoechoic region of fluid *anterior* to the descending thoracic aorta.

Answer choice *a* is consistent with severe sepsis, with the echocardiogram showing hyperdynamic left ventricular and intravascular volume depletion, evidenced by the decreased diameter of the inferior vena cava and inspiratory collapse. Choice *b* is consistent with a large pulmonary embolus with clinical and echocardiographic findings of right ventricular overload. The McConnell sign was initially thought to be specific for pulmonary embolism; however, this has since been disputed. The sign indicates hypokinesia of the mid–free wall of the right ventricle with normal apical movement. Choice *c* illustrates a pericardial friction rub; however, the echocardiographic findings show fluid in the pleural space, which is identified by hypoechoic fluid posterior to the descending thoracic aorta. Right atrial collapse during less than 33% of the cardiac cycle is relatively nonspecific for cardiac tamponade. Choice *e* is consistent with dilated cardiomyopathy and heart failure. The echocardiogram shows 4-chamber dilatation with hypoechoic material (ie, blood) inside the heart.

19. Answer b.

The key is to identify the set of results with an increased ratio of total calcium to ionized calcium of at least 2.5 along with a decreased bicarbonate level. In answer choice *b*, the ratio of total calcium to ionized calcium is 3, which is suggestive of citrate toxicity in this patient with liver cirrhosis who probably has decreased citrate metabolism. Albumin correction for total calcium levels was not applied in the studies that reported an association of citrate toxicity with a total calcium to ionized calcium ratio of 2.5 or more (NDT Plus. 2009;2[6]:439-47) or of 2.4 or more (Crit Care. 2012 Aug 22;16[4]:R162). The citrate infusion should be decreased to avoid complications from low ionized calcium levels, such as cardio-vascular instability or seizures.

20. Answer a.

Pituitary apoplexy is usually associated with diabetes mellitus, hypertension, sickle cell disease, and head trauma. An association with hyperthyroidism has not been described.

21. Answer e.

For critically ill patients with influenza, a prolonged course (>5 days) of oselta-mivir is recommended. Corticosteroids have no benefit in influenza pneumonitis and may be harmful. Broad-spectrum antibiotic therapy should be continued until microbiology results are available because secondary bacterial pneumonia may occur (the most common pathogens are *Staphylococcus aureus, Streptococcus pneumoniae,* and *Streptococcus pyogenes*). Intravenous zanamivir should be considered if patients have a documented oseltamivir resistance, are severely immunocompromised, and carry a high suspicion for oseltamivir resistance or if gastric absorption of oseltamivir is a concern. Critically ill patients may decompensate despite receiving oseltamivir, but those situations have rarely been attributed to resistance.

22. Answer c.

The patient has rapidly evolving skin lesions, and because of her immunosuppressed state, mucormycosis is very high in the differential diagnosis. The rapid evolution of the lesions could result from a bacterial skin infection, so broad-spectrum antibiotics should be initiated. Antifungals, such as amphotericin B liposomal complex to treat mucormycosis, should be started, and a surgical consultation for prompt débridement must be sought because patients with mucormycosis have high morbidity and mortality.

23. Answer a.

The electrocardiographic rhythm strip is interpreted as torsades de pointes. Immediate management of this dysrhythmia includes optimizing electrolytes and removing QT-prolonging medications. Administering magnesium 2 g intravenously is beneficial in terminating torsades de pointes in patients who have congenital or acquired prolonged QT. The exact mechanism as to why magnesium is so effective in aborting this rhythm is not fully understood but is thought to involve the blockage of sodium or calcium channels.

24. Answer c.

Anticardiolipin antibody and lupus anticoagulant (or lupus inhibitor) are 2 of the primary antibodies that interfere with platelet membrane phospholipids. Therefore, disturbance will lead to platelet aggregation and thrombosis. Lupus anticoagulant often leads to a prolonged activated partial thromboplastin time. Ferritin levels are often elevated as much as 800 to 1,000 times in acute presentations, and antiphospholipid syndrome is considered one of the hyperferritinemic syndromes. β_2-Glycoprotein 1 antibody test results will be elevated and are less common than anticardiolipin antibody but may be more specific in the diagnosis of antiphospholipid syndrome. This test should not be confused with the β_2-microglobulin test, which is used to identify a tumor marker in multiple myeloma, leukemia, and lymphomas. It is also used after kidney transplant to follow patients for signs of rejection or damage to glomeruli or tubules.

25. Answer d.

Transfusion-related acute lung injury (TRALI) is a form of acute respiratory distress syndrome (ARDS) that occurs within minutes or up to 6 hours after transfusion in the absence of other causes. The risk of TRALI is higher with plasma and platelet transfusion, but TRALI may occur with any type of blood product. Patients with TRALI commonly have other features of systemic inflammatory response, such as fever or hypotension. Therefore, although TRALI should be considered in the differential diagnosis, it seems less likely. In this young patient with no history of cardiovascular disorder or risk factors, the possibility of volume overload or perioperative myocardial infarction is very low. Aspiration-related lung injury is also unlikely in the absence of aspiration. The temporal relation of witnessed laryngospasm followed by relief of upper airway obstruction strongly points to negative-pressure pulmonary edema.

26. Answer c.

This patient has diabetic ketoacidosis (DKA), which was likely precipitated by a gastrointestinal tract illness and the holding of her home insulin. Most patients with DKA present with profound dehydration because of glucosuria. This patient's dehydration is exacerbated by emesis and decreased oral intake. Initial treatment should focus on volume resuscitation with crystalloids. Because potassium shifts out of cells during metabolic acidosis, serum potassium levels are usually normal. Even if they have normal levels of serum potassium, patients likely have a whole-body potassium deficit. This patient has a low potassium level, so a severe potassium deficit should be anticipated and parenteral replacement of potassium should be initiated before an insulin infusion is started; otherwise, severe hypokalemia may ensue.

Abdominal pain is common during DKA, and although a primary abdominal disorder is possible, initial treatment should focus on restoring the intravascular volume status and treating electrolyte abnormalities. Although an arterial line may be useful for monitoring this patient's hemodynamics and obtaining frequent blood samples, it is not the best next step. Before the patient is discharged from the intensive care unit, an endocrinology consultation may be helpful to provide assistance with transitioning to a subcutaneous insulin regimen and outpatient recommendations, but it is not necessary with this acute disorder.

27. Answer d.

The presence of acute electrolyte disturbances (hyperkalemia, hyperphosphatemia, and hypocalcemia) along with hyperuricemia shortly after the initiation of cancer therapy (chemotherapy, radiotherapy, or biologic agents) is consistent with tumor lysis syndrome (TLS). The Cairo-Bishop laboratory and clinical criteria are used to establish the diagnosis of TLS. Although atrial fibrillation with rapid ventricular response is often associated with hemodynamic changes and may have contributed to this patient's poor renal function, the underlying cause of both the onset of atrial fibrillation and the acute kidney injury could be the acute and severe electrolyte abnormalities of TLS (hyperkalemia, hyperuricemia, and hypocalcemia). Rituximab has not been shown to cause acute interstitial nephritis; in fact, rituximab has been used to treat tubular interstitial nephritis associated with immunoglobulin G4-related systemic disease (Nephrol Dial Transplant. 2011 Jun;26[6]:2047-50). This patient does have physical examination and chest radiographic findings that are suggestive of pneumonia, and other findings suggest possible sepsis, but the laboratory values can be explained better by TLS. Leukemia-induced interstitial nephritis from high lysosome levels leads to potassium wasting and hypokalemia, not hyperkalemia as in this patient.

28. Answer c.

The patient likely has severe systemic vasculitis that involves her kidneys and lungs and is now complicated by diffuse alveolar hemorrhage (DAH). DAH is a clinical syndrome characterized by hypoxia and alveolar infiltrates and usually anemia and hemoptysis. Commonly an underlying antineutrophil cytoplasmic autoantibody–associated vasculitis or connective tissue disease is present.

Bronchoscopy should be performed to rule out infection and rule in alveolar hemorrhage. High-dose glucocorticoids and usually cyclophosphamide or rituximab should be started early for this life-threatening condition if clinical suspicion is high for DAH caused by a systemic vasculitis, even if test results for infectious causes are still pending. Any underlying coagulopathy should be reversed, but for this patient, who has a normal international normalized ratio, administering fresh frozen plasma is not the best answer. Plasmapheresis is indicated in Goodpasture syndrome but is only investigational for other causes of DAH, so glucocorticoids should still be given first. Although this patient may need dialysis, the refractory hypoxia requires urgent treatment targeted at the underlying cause. The echocardiogram does not indicate fluid overload, so diuresis would likely be of little benefit in the presence of alveolar hemorrhage.

29. Answer c.

The pathogenesis of paraneoplastic neurologic syndrome (PNS) is related to an autoimmune response and was understood with the discovery of multiple autoantibodies. By definition, a PNS is an effect of cancer that is not directly caused by tumor and metastasis. Other causes, including infections and metabolic derangements, must be ruled out.

30. Answer d.

This patient fulfills multiple criteria for severe-complicated *Clostridium difficile* infection (CDI): severe sepsis, hypotension, intensive care unit admission, and ileus. Intravenous vancomycin is not indicated in the treatment of intestinal CDI. Fecal microbiota transplantation is reserved for patients with recurrent CDI and is rarely used for patients with unresponsive severe CDI. Intravenous immunoglobulin has been used in cases of severe, refractory, or recurrent CDI, but the success rates are limited. Fidaxomicin is a macrolide antibiotic with response rates similar to those of vancomycin, and its role in severe-complicated CDI is yet to be defined.

The role of surgical therapy in CDI is advancing and should be considered for patients with severe-complicated CDI before colonic perforation or toxic megacolon develops. Surgical intervention can be lifesaving for patients with septic shock and should be considered early because perioperative mortality increases considerably if the leukocyte count increases to $50,000 \times 10^9/L$ or the serum lactate level increases to 5 mmol/L. Delaying surgery in patients with severe-complicated CDI is associated with adverse outcomes, including death. Hence, a surgical consultation should be sought early if a patient has sepsis, megacolon, or failure of maximal medical therapy (Mayo Clin Proc. 2012 Nov;87[11]:1106-17).

31. Answer c.

In the initial stages of shock, crystalloid fluid boluses are used. The World Health Organization guidelines recommend gelatin-based, dextran-based, or starch-based colloids when a poor response is noted. Pleural effusions do not generally require chest tube placement because the fluid is a transudate and the use of chest tubes carries the risk of significant bleeding. Blood products such as packed red blood cells or fresh whole blood have been recommended for hemorrhagic complications. Little evidence exists to support the use of prophylactic platelet or plasma transfusions. There is no evidence to support the use of corticosteroids, intravenous immunoglobulin, or recombinant factor VII concentrate.

32. Answer e.

This patient has recurrent fever with negative results from an infectious disease workup. A patient with localized cellulitis is unlikely to present with fever and features of persistent sepsis for several months. Elevated serum triglyceride and ferritin levels, bone marrow biopsy with evidence of erythrophagocytosis, and leukopenia are features of hemophagocytic syndrome and may suggest a diagnosis. Confirmation requires further evidence, such as a high level of soluble interleukin 2 receptor. Secondary causes of hemophagocytosis, such as atypical infections, should also be evaluated (eg, *Histoplasma*, viruses, and autoimmune disease).

33. Answer b.

A third-generation cephalosporin should be initiated because this patient's polymorphonuclear neutrophil count is more than 250/mcL, and he may have spontaneous bacterial peritonitis (SBP). Patients with culture-negative neutrocytic ascites have symptoms and mortality rates that are similar to those of patients with SBP (Hepatology. 2009 Jun;49[6]:2087-107). When follow-up ascitic fluid is obtained, about 34% of these patients have positive cultures (Hepatology. 2009 Jun;49[6]:2087-107).

34. Answer b.

Polyarteritis nodosa is an antinuclear antibody–negative vasculitis that commonly affects medium-sized to small arteries. The kidney is the organ most commonly affected by vasculitis besides the gastrointestinal tract, skin, and nervous system.

Usually patients are in the third or fourth decade of life and present with systemic symptoms such as fatigue, arthralgias, weight loss, or fever. They may also present with peripheral neuropathy or mononeuritis multiplex and skin nodules, purpura, livedo, testicular infarction, or primary renal involvement (like the patient in this question). Associations with hepatitis B virus infection have been described in 30% to 40% of patients. No specific diagnostic criteria exist. The diagnosis is confirmed with renal angiography, which shows characteristically numerous microaneurysms in the renal artery, or with biopsy of the affected organs (eg, skin or nerve). Treatment with corticosteroids alone or in combination with cyclophosphamides helps to induce remission.

35. Answer e.

The patient has Guillain-Barré syndrome that was not initially recognized because of the respiratory deterioration secondary to the aspiration event from the associated dysphagia. When her sedation was stopped, the full clinical syndrome became apparent. Areflexia, flaccid quadraplegia, a normal creatine kinase level, and reduced compound muscle action potential amplitudes can be seen both with critical illness neuromyopathy (CINM) and with Guillain-Barré syndrome; however, isolated cranial neuropathies do not occur with CINM. The patient's cranial nerve palsy and the slowed conduction velocities on the nerve conduction study are clues to the diagnosis of Guillain-Barré syndrome (Muscle Nerve. 2013 Mar;47[3]:452-63. Epub 2013 Feb 6).

36. Answer d.

This patient is presenting with neuroleptic malignant syndrome (NMS) secondary to her long-standing use of high-dose quetiapine and concurrent use of prochlorperazine for her migraine exacerbation. Her altered mental status and rigidity are typical features of NMS on examination, and the clear red urine in her Foley catheter drainage bag may be consistent with myoglobinuria from rhabdomyolysis. Most concerning, however, is her dysautonomia and respiratory distress with hypoxemic and hypercapnic respiratory failure from her chest wall rigidity and possible aspiration. The administration of dantrolene, bromocriptine, and possibly bicarbonate is indicated in her situation, but the best immediate action would be endotracheal intubation and mechanical ventilation for stabilization. The administration of antihypertensives in a patient who has dysautonomia from NMS should be done cautiously with low doses of agents that are quickly metabolized (Neurol Clin. 2004 May;22[2]:389-411).

37. Answer b.

N-acetylcysteine (NAC) therapy would be the best next step in the management of this patient. Acetaminophen poisoning is the most likely diagnosis given her history and clinical presentation, which suggest stage 2 acetaminophen poisoning. Although NAC has maximal efficacy within 8 hours after acetaminophen ingestion, the prognosis may improve even if NAC is administered within 48 hours after ingestion (Crit Care Clin. 2012 Oct;28[4]:499-516). Both oral and intravenous NAC therapies have been shown to be equally efficacious in preventing liver failure when administered early. Direct comparisons are lacking, and the route of administration may be dictated by drug availability and the patient's ability to take medication orally (West J Emerg Med. 2013 May;14[3]:218-26).

Cimetidine (answer choice *a*) has been shown to be beneficial for acetaminophen poisoning in animal models, but data for humans are not convincing.

Serum acetaminophen levels (choice *c*) are useful to guide therapy in the first 24 hours after ingestion. This patient has been symptomatic for 36 hours, so acetaminophen levels would not help guide therapy according to a nomogram, although increased levels can be used to confirm the diagnosis. There is no indication to delay possible lifesaving therapy to obtain a result that would not rule out the most important differential diagnosis.

Lactulose therapy (choice *d*) can be used to manage hepatic encephalopathy. Although it would not be the next step, it may be indicated later in the clinical course. It is better to treat the cause of hyperammonemia rather than the increased serum ammonia level.

Serum ethanol levels (choice *e*) may help in the diagnosis of acute alcoholic hepatitis. However, this patient's symptoms started 36 hours ago, so the blood alcohol concentration would be decreasing by now. The ratio of aspartate aminotransferase to alanine aminotransferase and the absolute values of the aminotransferases do not support the diagnosis of alcoholic hepatitis (in which the ratio is generally >2:1 and the levels generally are not >500 U/L).

38. Answer e.

Hyperreflexia, muscle rigidity, focal neurologic deficit, and decerebrate posturing have all been reported as manifestations of severe hepatic encephalopathy. Focal neurologic deficit and decerebrate posturing are less commonly reported and may indicate more advanced or severe neurologic injury. Early recognition and assessment for other causes is essential.

39. Answer a.

Failure to exclude all confounding factors is a hazardous pitfall during the clinical examination to establish brain death. For this patient, it would have been essential to check the serum alcohol level given the history of alcoholism and thus the possibility that she may have been intoxicated when she fell. In addition, evaluation of serum electrolytes, liver function, kidney function, and blood glucose is also essential. A reliable neurologic examination cannot be performed at a core temperature of 33°C; the patient should be warmed to normothermia before proceeding with a clinical examination. She had received midazolam and vecuronium during intubation, and thus the lingering effects of these medications cannot be excluded. With all these confounding factors, it is best to defer examination for brain death in the emergency department. Occasionally, patients have stereotypical reflex motor responses to noxious stimulation in the extremities. The presence of these reflexes does not indicate any residual functioning of the brainstem or the cerebral hemispheres because they are usually mediated through the spinal cord (Neurology. 1995 May;45[5]:1012-4). Thus, they do not necessarily preclude the declaration of brain death.

40. Answer c.

Venovenous extracorporeal membrane oxygenation (ECMO) is the therapy of choice for adults with isolated respiratory failure, whereas venoarterial ECMO is the therapy of choice for isolated cardiac failure or for cardiopulmonary failure. Neuromuscular blockade (answer choice *a*) may be used in early ECMO if patients continue to have severe hypoxia despite the initiation of ECMO. As oxygenation improves, neuromuscular blockade should be discontinued regardless of the duration of ECMO, and certainly it should be discontinued before weaning from ECMO. Mechanical ventilation (choice *b*) is frequently continued for patients receiving ECMO, with lung-protective strategies including higher positive end-expiratory pressure (>10 cm H_2O) and plateau pressure less than 30 cm H_2O (ideally <25 cm H_2O), to prevent both ventilator-associated lung injury and lung collapse. At this time, there is no evidence that antimicrobial prophylaxis (choice *d*) prevents central line–associated infections in these patients; therefore, guidelines do not recommend this strategy for prevention of infection. Mechanical ventilation for more than 7 days (choice *e*) is considered a relative contraindication for ECMO initiation (according to the current Extracorporeal Life Support Organization guidelines) because of poorer outcomes with longer ventilation before starting ECMO therapy.

41. Answer c.

In this patient with a history of intravenous drug abuse, endocarditis is a potential cause of acute mitral regurgitation. A systolic murmur may be absent in 30% of patients with moderate or severe mitral regurgitation. Electrocardiographic findings may be normal or nonspecific. Although cardiac catheterization would establish the diagnosis of acute mitral regurgitation, echocardiography is preferred because of the lack of risks and the feasibility of obtaining this test. Additionally, echocardiography would allow for determination of the mechanism of mitral regurgitation. Computed tomography would further characterize the bilateral infiltrates but is not preferred over echocardiography for establishing the diagnosis of acute mitral regurgitation.

42. Answer d.

This patient is displaying signs and symptoms consistent with bowel infarction. Although the exact cause of the ischemia cannot be determined from the information provided, the likely causes include stent occlusion (eg, in-stent thrombosis), stent migration, or embolization. Surgical intervention is the definitive treatment of bowel ischemia or infarction in this patient who is in shock. Although abdominal computed tomography with a contrast agent (choice *a*) would help with diagnosis, surgical intervention is of utmost importance.

43. Answer a.

From the information presented, periengraftment respiratory distress syndrome is suggested and empirical therapy with high-dose methylprednisolone should be initiated. The patient has had neutropenic fever, diarrhea, dyspnea, bilateral infiltrates, and rash during the engraftment period with no evidence of cardiogenic pulmonary edema. A favorable response to intravenous corticosteroids would confirm the diagnosis.

Furosemide (choice *b*) may be helpful with pulmonary edema due to volume overload. In cardiogenic pulmonary edema, chest radiography typically shows fluid in the fissures and cardiomegaly. The brain natriuretic peptide level is expected to be elevated. A history of receiving a large volume of fluids and blood products may also be present.

Diffuse alveolar hemorrhage can occur during the engraftment period (median onset, 11-24 days) of both allogenic and autologous transplants. Treatment is with intravenous corticosteroids, and most patients require mechanical ventilation. The diagnosis is confirmed with bronchoalveolar lavage (choice *c*) showing progressively bloodier return from separate subsegmental bronchi or more than 40% hemosiderin-laden alveolar macrophages. Approximately one-third of patients with periengraftment respiratory distress syndrome also have diffuse alveolar hemorrhage.

The median onset of idiopathic pneumonia syndrome is between 21 and 87 days. Treatment includes supportive care and treatment of infection. Lung biopsy (choice *d*) may show diffuse alveolar damage, pneumonia, and interstitial lymphocytic inflammation.

Continuing the current management (choice *e*) would likely lead to worsening respiratory distress, a need for mechanical ventilation, and additional invasive diagnostic tests.

44. Answer d.

The patient likely has rib fractures (which are often missed with plain radiography) with underlying lung contusion. Limiting intravenous fluids prevents worsening of pulmonary edema in a patient with rib fractures and underlying lung contusion. Additionally, computed tomography of the chest would provide a better understanding of the extent of lung contusion and would be useful for diagnosing an occult pneumothorax missed with plain radiography. At this point, however, there is no indication of a pneumothorax or hemothorax, which would make chest tube insertion (choice *a*) unnecessary. Also, prophylactic chest tube insertion for rib fractures is not supported by the literature. With a normal mediastinum and cardiac silhouette on the chest radiograph, normal pulse pressure, and no other clinical signs of aortic dissection or cardiac tamponade, diagnostic or therapeutic interventions for these conditions (choices *b* and *e*) would not be warranted. The right mid lung infiltrate is unlikely to be secondary to aspiration pneumonitis (choice *c*) given that the patient's Glasgow Coma Scale score is 15 and there is no history of altered consciousness.

45. Answer e.

The appropriate dose of thyroid hormone replacement has not been well established, and evidence for treatment protocols are lacking. Myxedema is a potentially fatal condition that requires a multifaceted aggressive approach. Triiodothyronine has a rapid onset of action. If ileus is present, the oral route for treatment is not recommended because of concerns about intestinal function.

46. Answer b.

Bleeding time is uncommonly used and, as a test of platelet function, would not assist in making this diagnosis. All the other tests would be indicated to aid the diagnosis.

47. Answer b.

Ultrasonography is a portable, reliable tool for diagnosing or excluding pneumothorax. Pneumothorax is ruled out by the presence of lung sliding (a regular rhythmic movement synchronized with respiration that occurs between the parietal and visceral pleura), B lines (hyperechoic vertical artifacts that arise from the pleura), or lung point (subtle rhythmic movement of the visceral pleura on the parietal pleura with cardiac oscillations) (Crit Care Med. 2007 May;35[5 Suppl]:S250-61). The absence of lung sliding does not rule in pneumothorax, and it can be seen in various conditions, including acute respiratory distress syndrome, atelectasis, and pleural symphysis (Crit Care Med. 2007 May;35[5 Suppl]:S250-61). However, the abolished lung sliding can be diagnostic in the appropriate clinical context. The figure, an M-mode image of the left anterior pleura, shows multiple layers of horizontal lines. They are called the stratosphere sign, and, in M-mode ultrasonography, indicate the nonsliding pleura and lung parenchyma (Crit Care Med. 2007 May;35[5 Suppl]:S250-61). This sign is highly suggestive of pneumothorax in this previously healthy patient who sustained blunt chest trauma. He is presenting with signs and symptoms suggestive of tension pneumothorax, including tachycardia, hypotension, diminished breath sounds, and an increased oxygen requirement. A needle thoracostomy should be performed.

48. Answer c.

Despite a lack of evidence, double-dose oseltamivir therapy (150 mg twice daily) and a longer duration of therapy (>10 days) are recommended. The largest multicenter trial was in Southeast Asia during the 2009 H1N1 influenza virus pandemic: When double-dose therapy was compared with standard-dose therapy, no difference was found in intensive care unit length of stay, duration of mechanical ventilation, clearance of virus, or mortality.

49. Answer b.

This is a classic presentation of Dressler syndrome or late pericarditis post–cardiac injury syndrome. It is a form of immune-mediated pericarditis that usually occurs 4 to 6 weeks after cardiac injury. The most accepted theory is that cardiac injury releases previously concealed cardiac antigen and induces the formation of autoantibody against pericardium cells and local inflammation. Hence, Dressler syndrome occurs after acute coronary syndrome (ACS), myocarditis, and pericardiotomy. It is self-limited and characterized by fever, chest pain, and pericardial rub and is often treated successfully with nonsteroidal anti-inflammatory drugs.

Choice *a* describes viral myocarditis, which is unrelated to a recent infarction and often occurs with findings of acute heart failure. Choice *c* is the histologic description of ACS, which does not usually present with fever or pericardial rub, and the electrocardiogram (ECG) usually shows no PR interval changes. Choice *d* explains the underlying mechanism of esophageal spasm, which can occur with severe substernal chest pain relieved with nitroglycerin. However, there are no ECG changes, fever, or presence of a pericardial rub. Choice *e* explains the pathophysiology of costochondritis, which is a frequent cause of pain; however, it is not related to auscultatory or electrical findings, so this diagnosis is unlikely.

50. Answer c.

Desaturation is occurring, and the patient requires supplemental oxygen. His vocal cords were not visualized and he has a difficult airway. First, you must improve his oxygen saturation and then work with others on how to approach his airway safely. Never be too proud to call for help in an emergency. If you cannot successfully intubate the patient by using advanced techniques (fiberoptic intubation), a surgical airway is certainly an option that should be considered—but not this early. The changing of blades or attempting videolaryngoscopic intubation is unlikely to improve visualization given his significant oropharyngeal edema.

Index

Page numbers followed by *b, f,* or *t* indicate boxes, figures, or tables, respectively.

AAV. *see* antineutrophil cytoplasmic antibody
  (ANCA)–associated vasculitis
abdominal pain
  case presentation, 158–159
  in diabetic ketoacidosis, 269
  diffuse, 32–35, 33*t*
  in spontaneous renal artery dissection, 158–161
acetabular fracture, left, 58–59
acetaminophen overdose, 37–39, 38*f*, 171–173, 273
  acute liver failure secondary to, 170–172
  case presentations, 36–37, 37*t*, 170–171
  management of, 172–173
acetylsalicylic acid (aspirin)
  drug absorption, 43
  overdose, 42, 263
acid-base disturbances
  alcohol-related ketoacidosis, 263
  diabetic ketoacidosis, 118–120, 119*t*, 120–121,
    268–269
  high anion gap metabolic acidosis, 37–39
  in salicylate toxicity, 45
activated charcoal, 45–46
acute coronary syndrome
  case presentation, 225–226, 226*f*
  cocaine abuse related to, 225–227, 226*f*
acute eosinophilic pneumonia, 23–24, 261–262
  case presentation, 22–23
  diagnostic criteria for, 24
  therapy for, 24
acute kidney injury
  case presentation, 26

CRRT for, 86
acute liver failure secondary to acetaminophen
    overdose, 170–172
acute lung injury, transfusion-related (TRALI), 268
acute mitral regurgitation, 191–193
  case presentation, 190–191, 191*f*
  functional, 191–192
  management of, 192–193
  organic, 191–192
acute myeloid leukemia, 70–72
acute myocardial infarction, 49. *see also* myocardial
    infarction
acute pancreatitis, 32–33
  complications of, 33
  secondary to hypertriglyceridemia, 33–34,
    262–263
acute pulmonary edema, 199–200
acute pulmonary embolism, 60–61
acute renal failure, 124–128
  case presentations, 108–111, 124–125
acute respiratory distress syndrome, 219–221
  blastomycosis in, 20–21
  characterization of, 23
  differential diagnosis of, 23
  ECMO for, 184–188
  influenza A–associated, 96–97, 218–222
  influenza A–associated pandemic (2009-2010),
    96, 219
  management of, 21, 96–97, 219, 220
acute respiratory failure, 23
  differential diagnosis of, 23

acute respiratory failure (*Cont.*)
    ECMO for, 186
    in stem cell transplantation, 198–201
    in young smokers, 22–25
acute salicylate toxicity, 43–45
adenocarcinoma, metastatic, 2–3
adenoid cystic carcinoma, metastatic, 52–53
AEP. *see* acute eosinophilic pneumonia
airway emergencies
    algorithm for managing a difficult airway, 229,
        229*b*, 230–231*f*
    ball-valve obstruction, 115
    case presentation, 228
    difficult airway, 228–232, 278
    upper airway crisis, 114–117
alcoholic hepatitis, 273
alcohol-related ketoacidosis, 263
altered mental status, 166–169
alveolar hemorrhage, diffuse, 132–134, 269–270
    case presentation, 130–132, 131*f*, 132*t*
American Academy of Neurology: guidelines for
        determining brain death, 179
American College of Chest Physicians
        (ACCP): guidelines for thrombolytic therapy
        in massive pulmonary embolism, 61, 264
American Society of Anesthesiologists: algorithm
        for managing a difficult airway, 229, 229*b*,
        230–231*f*
amphotericin B deoxycholate, 21
amphotericin B lipid complex, 21
amyloidosis, 15, 15*f*
    AL, 15–16, 261
    liver failure in, 14–17, 261
    treatment of, 17
anesthesia
    excitement phase, 116
    laryngospasm during, 115
angioedema, laryngeal, 228–232
angiotensin-converting enzyme inhibitors, 228–232
anticardiolipin antibody, 268
anticholinergic toxicity, 168*t*
anticoagulation, 60–61
anti-GBM antibody disease, 133, 134
anti-GBM nephritis, 133, 134
antineutrophil cytoplasmic antibody (ANCA)–
        associated vasculitis (AAV), 133, 269–270
    relapse, 130–132, 131*f*, 132*t*
antiphospholipid syndrome, catastrophic, 111
    case presentation, 108–111, 109*t*
apical ballooning syndrome, 76
    characterization of, 77
    reverse apical ballooning syndrome, 74–78, 75*f*

ARDS. *see* acute respiratory distress syndrome
arrhythmias, 7, 267
    idioventricular, 260–261
aspirin (acetylsalicylic acid)
    drug absorption, 43
    overdose, 42, 263
ataxia, cerebellar, 137
atrial tachycardia, paroxysmal, 6–7
atropine, 116
autologous stem cell transplant. *see also* stem cell
        transplant
    case presentation, 198, 199*f*

bacterial peritonitis, spontaneous, 155–156, 271
    case presentation, 154–155
    diagnosis of, 155
    mortality rate, 156
    treatment of, 155, 156
ballooning, apical, 74–78
ball-valve obstruction, 115
Beck triad, 81
Bethesda assay, 212–213
biochemical abnormalities
    in CRRT, 87
    in DKA, 118–120, 119*t*
bioprosthetic valves, aortic, 70–71
bismuth subsalicylate (Pepto-Bismol), 42–43
Blastomyces dermatitidis, 20
blastomycosis, 20
    in ARDS, 20–21
    respiratory failure in, 18–20
    treatment of, 261
bleeding disorders, 210–213
    case presentation, 210–211
blood clots: clearing, 55
blood pressure
    high. *see* hypertension
    low. *see* hypotension
blurry vision, 108–111
bowel infarction, 275
brain death, 178–182
    case presentation, 178–179
    checklist for determining, 180*b*–181*b*
    determination of, 274
    guidelines for determining, 179
bronchoscopy, 55

CAPS. *see* catastrophic antiphospholipid syndrome
cardiac herniation, 67, 68
    diagnosis of, 69
    left-sided, 68
    management of, 69

cardiac injury, 277–278

cardiac tamponade, 2–3, 260, 266
    case presentation, 80–81, 81f
    clinical presentations of, 80–83
    diagnosis of, 81
    echocardiographic signs of, 82–83
    signs and symptoms of, 3
    ultrasonographic signs of, 3–4

cardiopulmonary resuscitation
    complications of, 214–217
    post-CPR flail chest, 202–205

cardiovascular disease, 7

cardiovascular injuries, post-CPR, 215

catastrophic antiphospholipid syndrome, 111
    case presentation, 108–111, 109t

catatonia, malignant, 168t

CDI. see Clostridium difficile infection

cerebellar ataxia, subacute, 137

charcoal, activated, 45–46

chest pain
    acute, 48
    case presentation, 225–226, 226f
    and respiratory distress, 190–193
    retrosternal, 48
    in reverse apical ballooning syndrome due to
        clonidine withdrawal, 74–76
    severe, 224–227

chest wall injuries
    post-CPR, 202–205
    treatment of, 204

chronic mitral regurgitation, 191, 192

chronic myeloid leukemia, 98–102

chronic obstructive lung disease, 36–37, 37t

Churg-Strauss syndrome, 133

cigarette smoking, 22–25

CINM. see critical illness neuromyopathy

cirrhosis: complications of, 154–157
    case presentation, 154–155

citrate toxicity, 86–87

clonidine withdrawal
    clinical manifestations of, 77
    reverse apical ballooning syndrome due to, 74–78

Clostridium difficile infection, 143–145
    case presentation, 142–143
    severe, 144
    severe-complicated, 144–145, 270–271

coagulation, 211, 212f

coagulation cascade defects, 211, 212–213

cocaine abuse
    ACS related to, 225–227, 226f
    case presentation, 225–226, 226f
    cocaine-induced ischemia, 226–227

COLD. see chronic obstructive lung disease

coma, 206–209
    case presentation, 206–207
    clinical presentation of, 207
    myxedema, 206–209

compartment syndrome, 166–167

continuous renal replacement therapy
    for acute kidney injury, 86
    case presentation, 84–85, 85t
    electrolyte abnormalities during, 84–88

coronary artery disease, 49

CPR. see cardiopulmonary resuscitation

critical illness myopathy, 163

critical illness neuromyopathy, 163–165, 272
    case presentation, 162–163
    diagnosis of, 164
    differential diagnosis of, 164
    management of, 164–165
    risk factors for, 163–164
    treatment options, 164

critical illness polyneuropathy, 163

CRRT. see continuous renal replacement therapy

crystalloids
    hypo-osmotic, 127
    for shock, 271
    for tumor lysis syndrome, 127

cytokine storm, 27, 199

DAH. see diffuse alveolar hemorrhage

death, brain, 178–182, 274

decerebrate posturing, 176

dengue hemorrhagic fever. see dengue shock
    syndrome

dengue shock syndrome, 148–149
    case presentation, 146–148
    critical phase, 148–149
    febrile phase, 148
    prevalence of, 148
    recovery phase, 149

dermatomyositis, 138

diabetes mellitus, type 2, 6–7
    case presentation, 118–120
    metabolic complications of, 120–121

diabetic ketoacidosis, 120–121, 268–269
    case presentation, 118–120, 119t
    laboratory findings in, 118–120, 119t
    management of, 121
    standardized protocol for, 118–119

diarrhea
    case presentation, 142–143
    complicated illness, 142–145
    infectious, 143–145

difficult airway, 278
  algorithm for managing a difficult airway, 229, 229b, 230–231f
  case presentation, 228
  treatment of, 228–232
diffuse abdominal pain, 32–35, 33t
diffuse alveolar hemorrhage, 132–134, 269–270
  case presentation, 130–132, 131f, 132t
diffuse pulmonary infiltrates, 130–134
disseminated histoplasmosis, 150–153
  case presentation, 150–152
disseminated intravascular coagulation, 70–72, 213
disseminated zygomycosis, 100
  case presentation, 98–99
DKA. see diabetic ketoacidosis
Dressler syndrome, 277–278
drug overdose
  acetaminophen, 36–39, 37t, 38f, 170–173, 273
  aspirin (acetylsalicylic acid), 42, 263
  over-the-counter, 36–40, 37t, 42–46
  salicylate, 42–46, 263
dyspnea, 2–5
  after autologous stem cell transplant, 198, 199f
  case presentation, 2–3
  hypoxia and diffuse pulmonary infiltrates in immunosuppression with vasculitis, 130–134
  in obesity-hypoventilation syndrome, 70–71
  in reverse apical ballooning syndrome due to clonidine withdrawal, 74–76
  in young smoker, 22–23

ECMO. see extracorporeal membrane oxygenation
edema, 2–5
  laryngeal angioedema, 228–232
  lower extremity, 2–3
  oropharyngeal, 278
  pulmonary, 62–64, 63f, 199–200, 265, 268
electrical problems, 6–8
  case presentation, 6–7
electrical storm, 7
electrolyte abnormalities
  during CRRT, 84–88
  in DKA, 118–120, 119t
embolism, pulmonary
  acute, 60–61
  anticoagulation for, 61
  case presentation, 58–59, 59f
  massive, 58–59, 59f, 60–61, 264
  therapy for, 60–61
encephalopathy, 174–176
  case presentation, 174–175
  hepatic, 174–176, 273

endocrine emergency, 118–120
engraftment syndrome, 199. see also periengraftment respiratory distress syndrome
eosinophilic granulomatosis, with polyangiitis, 133
eosinophilic pneumonia, acute, 23–24, 261–262
expiratory stridor, 115
extracorporeal life support, 186
extracorporeal membrane oxygenation, 186–187
  for acute respiratory failure, 186, 274
  for ARDS, 184–188, 220
  complications of, 187t
  contraindications to, 187t
  indications for, 186, 187t
  venoarterial, 185, 186–187, 274
  venovenous, 185, 186–187, 274
extubation failure, 62–65
  case presentation, 62–63

factor VIII inhibitors, 212–213
  case presentation, 210–211
  treatment of, 211, 213
fat pad aspiration, 15, 15f
fecal microbiota transplantation
  case presentation, 143
  for CDI, 144–145
ferritin, 268
fever, recurrent, 271
flail chest, 202–205
  case presentation, 202–203
  management of, 203–205
  post-CPR, 202–205
follicular lymphoma, 136–138
fractures
  acetabular, 58–59
  rib, 202–205, 214–217, 276

gas, portal venous, 194–197
γ-glutamyl cycle, 37–39, 38f
Goodpasture syndrome, 133
granulomatosis
  eosinophilic, with polyangiitis, 133
  with polyangiitis, 133
Guillain-Barré syndrome, 272

H1N1 influenza A virus infection, 96–97
  2009-2010 pandemic, 219, 220, 277
heart failure, right-sided, 66–69
hematopoietic stem cell transplant, 99–100
  mucormycosis after, 101
hemiparesis, left-sided, 80–81

hemodialysis
    indications for, 46
    for salicylate toxicity, 46
hemophagocytic lymphohistiocytosis, 152–153
    case presentation, 150–152
    diagnostic criteria for, 152
    treatment of, 152–153
hemophagocytosis, 151–152
hemophilia, acquired, 213
hemoptysis
    causes of, 54, 54*b*
    massive, 52–56, 53*f*, 264
hemorrhage
    diffuse alveolar, 130–132, 131*f*, 132–134, 132*t*,
        269–270
    persistent shock with hemorrhagic
        complications, 146–149
    subacute pituitary, 90–91, 91*f*
hepatic amyloidosis, 16
hepatic encephalopathy, 175–176, 273
    case presentation, 174–175
hepatitis, alcoholic, 273
herniation, cardiac, 67–69
hip, broken, 58–61
Histoplasma capsulatum, 153
histoplasmosis, disseminated, 150–153
HLH. *see* hemophagocytic lymphohistiocytosis
hydroxyurea, 73
hyperactivity, paroxysmal sympathetic, 168*t*
hypercalcemia, 87
hyperleukocytosis, 71–72, 265
hypernatremia, 87
hypertension, 10–13
    case presentation, 10–11
hypertensive crisis, 10
hyperthermia, malignant, 168*t*
hypertriglyceridemia
    acute pancreatitis in, 32–34, 262–263
    suggested therapeutic approaches for, 34
hypocalcemia, 87
hypokalemia, 87
hypomagnesemia, 87
hypo-osmotic crystalloids, 127
hypophosphatemia, 87
hypotension
    after broken hip, 58–61
    after left pneumonectomy, 66–69
hypothermia, 208
hypothyroidism, extreme, 206–209
hypoventilation, 207
    obesity-hypoventilation syndrome, 70–71

hypoxia
    after autologous stem cell transplant, 198, 199*f*
    case presentation, 130–132, 131*f*
    in immunosuppression with
        vasculitis, 130–134

ICU-acquired weakness, 163–165
    case presentation, 162–163
immunosuppression, 130–134
infection. *see also specific infections*
    with chronic myeloid leukemia, 98–102
    respiratory, 94–97
infectious diarrhea, 143–145
inferior vena cava plethora, 3–4
influenza, 96, 97
    risk factors for, 96
    therapy for, 97, 220–221, 267, 277
influenza A, 95–96
    2009-2010 pandemic, 219, 220, 277
    case presentation, 94–95
    H1N1, 96–97, 219, 220, 277
influenza A–associated ARDS
    2009-2010 pandemic, 96–97, 277
    case presentation, 218–219
    severe, 218–222
    therapy for, 96–97
injury
    post-CPR flail chest, 202–205
    post-CPR injuries, 202–205, 214–217
    transfusion-related acute lung injury
        (TRALI), 268
inspiratory stridor, 115
intensive care unit: weakness in, 162–165
intoxication
    acetaminophen overdose, 36–39, 37*t*, 38*f*,
        170–173, 273
    aspirin (acetylsalicylic acid)
        overdose, 42, 263
    over-the-counter overdose, 36–40, 37*t*, 42–46
    salicylate overdose, 42–46, 263
inverted takotsubo, 76
itraconazole, 21

jaw-thrust maneuver, 114, 116

ketoacidosis
    alcohol-related, 263
    diabetic, 118–120, 119*t*, 120–121, 268–269
kidneys
    acute kidney injury, 26, 86
    acute renal failure, 108–111, 124–128

Lambert-Eaton syndrome, 137
laryngeal angioedema, 228–232
    case presentation, 228
laryngospasm, 114–117
    during anesthesia, 115
    case presentation, 114
    risk factors for, 115
    strategies for limiting risk of, 116
    treatment of, 116–117
    types of, 115
laryngospasm notch, 116–117, 117f
late pericarditis post–cardiac injury syndrome,
        277–278
left acetabular fracture, 58–59
left pneumonectomy
    case presentation, 66–68
    hypotension and right-sided heart failure
        after, 66–69
left-sided cardiac herniation, 68
left-sided pleural effusion, 18–19, 19f, 81
leukemia
    acute myeloid, 70–72
    with blast crisis, 70–71
    chronic myeloid, 98–102
leukocytosis, 26
leukostasis, 70–73, 71t, 265
lidocaine, 116
liver failure, 14–17
    acute, 170–172
    in amyloidosis, 14–17, 261
    case presentations, 14–15, 170–171
    secondary to acetaminophen overdose, 170–172
    subacute, 14
    treatment of, 16–17
long QT syndrome, 105–106, 267
    acquired, 105–106
    case presentation, 104–105
    congenital, 105, 106
    pathophysiology of, 105–106
    therapy for, 106
    type 2, 104–105
lower extremity edema, 2–3
lung cancer, non–small cell, 80–81
lung disease, chronic obstructive, 36–37, 37t
lung injury
    post-CPR, 202–205, 214–217
    transfusion-related acute (TRALI), 268
lupus anticoagulant, 268
lupus inhibitor, 268
lymphohistiocytosis, hemophagocytic, 152–153
    case presentation, 150–152
lymphoma, follicular, 136–138

malignant catatonia, 168t
malignant hyperthermia, 168t
malignant mesothelioma, 66–68
mechanical ventilation, 139
meningeal carcinoma, 80–81
menstrual toxic shock syndrome, 29, 262
mental status, altered, 166–169
mesothelioma, malignant, 66–68
metabolic acidosis, high anion gap, 37–39
metabolic alkalosis, 87
metanephrines, fractionated, 261
methicillin-resistant Staphylococcus aureus, 27
methylprednisolone
    for acute eosinophilic pneumonia, 22–23, 24
    for CAPS and SLE, 110
    for DAH, 131, 134
methyl salicylate (wintergreen oil), 42–43
metronidazole
    for CDI, 144
    for diarrheal illness, 142
microscopic polyangiitis, 133
mitral regurgitation, 191–193
    acute, 190–193, 191f, 275
    case presentation, 190–191, 191f
    chronic, 191, 192
    papillary muscle rupture with, 263–264
M proteins, 29
mucormycosis, 99–101, 100f, 267
    case presentation, 98–99
    diagnosis of, 100–101
    treatment of, 101
multiple myeloma, 198, 199f
myeloid leukemia
    acute, 70–72
    chronic, 98–102
myocardial infarction
    acute, 49
    complications of, 49
    non–ST-segment elevation, 48
    post-MI complications, 48–51
    ST-segment elevation, 225–226, 226f
myocardial ischemia, cocaine-induced, 226–227
myopathy, critical illness, 163
myxedema coma, 207–209, 276
    case presentation, 206–207
    management of, 208–209
    pathognomonic features of, 207
    typical presentation of, 207
myxedema madness, 207

negative pressure pulmonary edema, 63–64,
        265, 268

nephritis, anti-GBM, 133, 134
neuraminidase inhibitors, 220–221
neuroendocrine tumors, 11, 12
neuroleptic malignant syndrome, 167–169, 272
    case presentation, 166–167
    differential diagnosis of, 168, 168t
    rigidity in, 166–169
    risk factors for, 167–168
    treatment of, 169
neuromuscular blockers, 218, 220, 221
neuromyopathy, critical illness, 163–165, 272
    case presentation, 162–163
    diagnosis of, 164
    differential diagnosis of, 164
    management of, 164–165
    risk factors for, 163–164
    treatment options, 164
neutrophil engraftment, 199
NMBs. *see* neuromuscular blockers
NMS. *see* neuroleptic malignant syndrome
noninvasive positive pressure ventilation
    (NIPPV), 139
non–small cell lung cancer, 80–81

obesity-hypoventilation syndrome, 70–71
occult pneumothorax
    definition of, 215
    secondary to CPR, 215–216
oropharyngeal edema, 278
oseltamivir, 220–221, 267, 277
ovarian cancer, metastatic, 266
    case presentation, 194, 195f
overdose
    acetaminophen, 36–39, 37t, 38f,
        170–173, 273
    aspirin (acetylsalicylic acid), 42, 263
    over-the-counter, 36–40, 37t, 42–46
    salicylate, 42–46, 263
over-the-counter overdose, 36–40, 42–46, 263
    case presentations, 36–37, 37t, 42
5-oxoproline (pyroglutamic acid) intoxication,
    37–39, 38f
    case presentation, 36–37, 37t

pain
    abdominal, 32–35, 33t, 158–161, 269
    chest pain, 48, 74–76, 190–193, 224–227
pancreatitis, acute, 32–34, 262–263
papillary muscle rupture, 263–264
paragangliomas
    diagnosis of, 12
    para-aortic, 10–11

parasympathetic, 11
sympathetic, 11
paraneoplastic neurologic syndrome, 136–140
    case presentation, 136–137
    diagnosis of, 138
    pathogenesis of, 137, 270
paroxysmal sympathetic hyperactivity, 168t
Pepto-Bismol (bismuth subsalicylate), 42–43
PERDS. *see* periengraftment respiratory distress
    syndrome
pericardial effusion
    evaluation of, 3–4
    with tamponade, 48, 81, 81f, 82
pericardiocentesis, ultrasound-guided, 3, 4
pericarditis, 277–278
periengraftment respiratory distress syndrome,
    199–200, 275–276
    case presentation, 198, 199f
peritonitis, spontaneous bacterial, 155–156
    case presentation, 154–155
pheochromocytomas, 11
    clinical presentation of, 12
    diagnosis of, 12
    surgical resection of, 12
pituitary apoplexy, 91–92, 267
    case presentation, 90–91, 91f
    diagnosis of, 92
pituitary hemorrhage, subacute, 90–91, 91f
platelet disorders, 211, 268
pleural effusion, left-sided, 18–19, 19f, 81
pneumatosis intestinalis, 196–197
    case presentation, 194, 195f
    etiology of, 196b, 197
    pathogenesis of, 197
pneumonectomy, left
    case presentation, 66–68
    hypotension and right-sided heart failure
        after, 66–69
pneumonia
    acute eosinophilic, 23–24, 261–262
    idiopathic syndrome, 276
pneumothorax
    occult, 215–216
    secondary to CPR, 214–217
    tension, 214–216, 277
    ultrasonography in, 277
PNS. *see* paraneoplastic neurologic syndrome
poisoning. *see* overdose
polyarteritis nodosa, 271
polyneuropathy, critical illness, 163
portal venous gas, 194–197
    case presentation, 194, 195f

prednisone
  for acute eosinophilic pneumonia, 24
  for acute respiratory failure, 23
  for ARDS, 21
  for DAH, 131
prone ventilation, 220
propofol, 116
Puerto Rico, 148
pulmonary artery compression, 67, 67f
pulmonary edema, 62–63, 63f
  acute, 199–200
  negative-pressure, 63–64, 265, 268
pulmonary embolism
  acute, 60–61
  anticoagulation for, 61
  case presentation, 58–59, 59f
  massive, 58–59, 59f, 60–61, 264
  therapy for, 60–61
pulmonary infiltrates, diffuse, 130–134
pulmonary injury
  post-CPR, 202–205, 214–217
  transfusion-related acute lung injury (TRALI), 268
pyroglutamic acid (5-oxoproline) intoxication,
      37–39, 38f
  case presentation, 36–37, 37t

renal artery dissection, spontaneous, 159–161
  case presentation, 158–159, 159f
renal failure, acute, 124–128
  case presentations, 108–111, 124–125
renal replacement therapy, continuous
  for acute kidney injury, 86
  case presentation, 84–85, 85t
  electrolyte abnormalities during, 84–88
respiratory distress
  ARDS, 96–97, 184–188, 218–222
  chest pain and, 190–193
  periengraftment syndrome, 198, 199–200, 199f,
      275–276
respiratory failure
  acute, 22–25, 198–201
  in blastomycosis, 18–20
  hypoxemic, 18–20
respiratory infection, 94–97
  case presentation, 94–95
resuscitation, cardiopulmonary
  complications of, 214–217
  post-CPR flail chest, 202–205
reverse apical ballooning syndrome, 74–78, 75f
rhabdomyolysis
  case presentation, 166–167
  treatment of, 169

rib fractures, 276
  case presentation, 202–203
  post-CPR, 202–205, 214–217
  surgical fixation of, 204
right innominate artery stent graft placement,
      52–53, 53f
right-sided heart failure, 66–69
rigidity, 166–169
rituximab, 131–132

salicylate overdose, 42–46, 263
  acid-base disturbances in, 45
  acute, 43–45
  case presentation, 42
  therapy for, 45–46
salicylates
  metabolic effects of, 42–43, 44f
  over-the-counter formulations, 42–43
SBP. see spontaneous bacterial peritonitis
septic shock mimic, 90–92
serotonin syndrome, 168t
shock, 26–30, 271
  case presentation, 26–27
  dengue shock syndrome, 146–149
  obstructive, 2–3
  persistent, with hemorrhagic complications,
      146–149
  recommendations for, 271
  septic shock mimic, 90–92
shortness of breath, 18–21
  case presentations, 2–3, 18–20
  dyspnea, 2–5, 22–23
  in reverse apical ballooning syndrome due to
      clonidine withdrawal, 74–76
  in young smoker, 22–23
SLE. see systemic lupus erythematosus
small-bowel obstruction, 118–120
smoking, 22–25
sodium bicarbonate, 46
somnolence, 207
spontaneous bacterial peritonitis, 155–156, 271
  case presentation, 154–155
  diagnosis of, 155
  mortality rate, 156
  treatment of, 155, 156
staphylococcal toxic shock syndrome, 28b, 29
Staphylococcus aureus, methicillin-resistant, 27
stem cell transplant
  acute respiratory failure in, 198–201
  for amyloidosis, 17
  autologous, 198, 199f
  case presentation, 198, 199f

stem cell transplant (*Cont.*)
    hematopoietic, 99–101
    mucormycosis after, 99–101
    pulmonary complications of, 200
stents, tracheal, 52–53, 53*f*
stratosphere sign, 277
streptococcal toxic shock syndrome, 27, 28*b*, 29
Streptococcus pyogenes, 27
stress cardiomyopathy, 76
stridor
    expiratory, 115
    inspiratory, 115
ST-segment elevation MI, 225–226, 226*f*
subacute cerebellar ataxia, 137
succinylcholine, 116
suicide attempts
    aspirin (acetylsalicylic acid) overdose, 42
    case presentation, 42
sympathetic hyperactivity, paroxysmal, 168*t*
sympathomimetic toxicity, 168*t*
systemic lupus erythematosus, 108–111, 109*t*

takotsubo cardiomyopathy, 76, 265–266
    clinical features of, 78
    inverted takotsubo, 76
    pathophysiology of, 76–77
tension pneumothorax, 277
    secondary to CPR, 214–217
    treatment of, 216
thoracic trauma, post-CPR, 202–205, 214–217
thrombocytopenia, 26
thrombolytic therapy
    for pulmonary embolism, 60–61, 264
    systemic, 61, 264
thrombotic microangiopathy, 111
thyroid replacement therapy, 207, 208–209, 276
thyroxine (T_4), 208–209
tongue swelling, 228
torsades de pointes, 104–106, 267
    case presentation, 104–105
toxic shock syndrome, 27, 29–30
    case presentation, 26–27
    diagnostic criteria for, 27, 28*b*
    menstrual, 29, 262
    staphylococcal, 28*b*, 29
    streptococcal, 27, 28*b*, 29
tracheal stents, 52–53, 53*f*
tracheal tumors, 52–53
TRALI. *see* transfusion-related acute lung injury
transfusion-related acute lung injury (TRALI), 268
transplantation
    fecal microbiota, 143, 144–145
    stem cell, 17, 99–101, 198–201, 199*f*

trauma, post-CPR thoracic, 202–205, 214–217
triglycerides. *see* hypertriglyceridemia
triiodothyronine (T_3), 208–209, 276
tumor lysis syndrome, 72, 125–127, 269
    Cairo-Bishop criteria for, 124–125, 126*b*
    case presentations, 70–71, 124–125
    pathophysiology of, 125, 126*f*
    prophylaxis of, 73
    risk factors for, 125
    spontaneous, 70–71
    treatment of, 127

ultrasonography
    in cardiac tamponade, 3–4
    in pneumothorax, 277
    stratosphere sign, 277
    swinging heart sign, 2–3
ultrasonographically guided
    pericardiocentesis, 2–4
upper airway crisis, 114–117
    case presentation, 114
    obstruction in laryngospasm, 114–117

vancomycin
    for CDI, 144
    for diarrheal illness, 142, 143
vasculitis
    ANCA–associated, 130–133, 131*f*, 132*t*, 269–270
    immunosuppression with, 130–134
    systemic, 271–272
ventilation
    mechanical, 139
    prone, 220
ventricular fibrillation, 7
ventricular free wall rupture, 49–51, 263–264
    case presentation, 48
    risk factors for, 49
    types of, 49–50
ventricular tachycardia
    refractory, 6–7
    sustained, 7
VFWR. *see* ventricular free wall rupture

weakness
    case presentation, 162–163
    ICU-acquired, 162–165
Wegener granulomatosis, 133
wintergreen oil (methyl salicylate), 42–43
withdrawal, clonidine
    clinical manifestations of, 77
    reverse apical ballooning syndrome due
        to, 74–78

women
    acetaminophen intoxication in, 36–39, 37*t*, 38*f*
    diffuse abdominal pain in 45-year-old woman,
        32–35, 33*t*
World Health Organization (WHO): guidelines for
    influenza therapy, 221

young smokers: acute respiratory
    failure in, 22–25

zanamivir, 220
zygomycosis, disseminated, 100
    case presentation, 98–99